He Said, "You Have Prostate Cancer"

He Said, "You Have Prostate Cancer"

This is the book the author couldn't find when he needed it—His journal of what came next.

STANLEY K SANDAGE

Writers Club Press

San Jose New York Lincoln Shanghai

He Said, "You Have Prostate Cancer"
This is the book the author couldn't find when he needed it—His journal of what came next.

Writers Club Press
an imprint of iUniverse, Inc.

For information address:
iUniverse, Inc.
5220 S. 16th St., Suite 200
Lincoln, NE 68512
www.iuniverse.com

ISBN: 0-595-23510-7

Printed in the United States of America

Dedicated to the cancer patients I met along the way.

May those who follow have more humane options

Contents

INTRODUCTION

In 1997, I was diagnosed with prostate cancer. I was devastated. After additional tests, I had discussions with specialists about a variety of treatment options. Then I learned, to my surprise, that I was expected to make the life or death treatment choice myself.

I was a 72 year old retired business man. I am not a doctor. I knew the fear of cancer—but I didn't know anything about a prostate. Asking a neophyte to make a medical decision of such magnitude seemed absurd. I realized then that I had no recourse—I would have to educate myself. My doctor agreed that it would be OK to delay my treatment decision for a few months.

My initial instinct was to find a reliable book that would include the latest medical advances in treating prostate cancer. I soon learned that recently published books on this subject didn't exist. And later, I was to make the astounding discovery that within the last several decades, there had been an almost total medical void of significant advances in treating prostate cancer.

This book is almost a five-year journal of my life after I learned that I had prostate cancer. It includes sharing what I learned during the frustrating process of trying to educate myself, making my decision, undergoing treatment, post-treatment experiences, plus my accompanying emotional ups and downs. Its purpose is to provide a prospective prostate cancer patient with the book I couldn't find when I needed it.

Years ago when I was scheduled for a heart bypass, before it became popular, I was obviously uptight and nervous. A fellow employee, who had recently undergone such an operation, shared his experience with me. His visit calmed me to such an extent that my surgeon drafted me to visit his pre-surgery patients, which I did for the next ten years. People who have some familiarity with what to expect make better patients. Hopefully this book will substitute for my visit. I hope it will ease your load along the way.

For obvious reasons I have substituted fictitious names for the real names of my doctors. Also, after the early pages, I have abbreviated these most frequently used words:

PC—for Prostate Cancer

PSA—for Prostate-specific Antigen

AGMC—for Akron General Medical Center

1

A POSITIVE BIOPSY

(FEB. 1997)

We purchased a new Camry in 1991. It was in early 1996 when I noticed what I thought was some superficial rust around the rear wheel wells. I used some rubbing compound which seemed to solve the problem. I never gave it another thought until later in the fall when I noticed that rust had returned with a vengeance. When I finally drove into a body shop to get an appraisal, I got a big surprise. The manager showed me in the owner's manual where it clearly provides an unlimited warranty against "corrosion perforation" for a five-year period. Had I reviewed my warranty when I first noticed some rust in 1996, I would have been covered. I not only would have been entitled to the repair at no cost, but the warranty on the repair itself would have been extended for another 5 years. Negligence can be very costly.

For the past several years I have been taking medication to control my cholesterol and I have my blood tested every six months to check its effectiveness and to be assured that it isn't damaging my liver. On February 5, 1997, when I made my routine stop at my doctor's office to have blood drawn, it occurred to me that I hadn't had a prostate test recently. I asked the technician to draw additional blood for a PSA test, which she did. PSA is the abbreviation for *prostate-specific antigen*, a substance produced only by the prostate. A PSA test measures the level of PSA in the bloodstream. Very little PSA escapes from a healthy prostate, but certain prostatic conditions, including cancer, can cause larger amounts of PSA to leak into the bloodstream (malignant tissue produces 10 times more PSA than does benign tissue). The PSA test, discovered around 1989, has become the "best measurement" of determining the possibility of having cancer of the prostate.

Two days later I received a call from my doctor's office asking me to stop in the next day. All she would tell me was that there was a high reading on one of my tests. This call triggered all kinds of warning signals, which made for a long sleepless night.

When I walked into that office the following day, I was quickly whisked into the room of a nurse practitioner (my doctor wasn't available on such short notice). What she told me, in her somber but professional voice, would impact my life more than any message I had ever received. She told me that my PSA measured 10 ng/ml (Nanograms per Milliliter) which was more than double a normal reading. My records revealed that my last PSA test had been in 1994 and it had measured 4.8 ng/ml. I vaguely remembered that my doctor had referred to that reading at the time as a "high normal" for my age and he didn't voice much concern. Now it measured 10. That's when the realization struck me that, after 72 years, I was probably facing the most significant and most terrifying problem of my life, and one which I would have very little ability to control. Why wasn't I referred to a urologist in 1994? Why didn't I follow through myself, and get retested in 1995, or 1996! Now I was facing a problem that certainly would have been less ominous had it been dealt with earlier. That's when I realized the irony: just as my car was now rusting away because I was careless and didn't take immediate action, now my body would likely suffer a similar fate for the same reason.

Five days later, as soon as I could get an appointment; my wife Peg and I walked into the office of Dr. Callon, a urologist. He was professional and direct—and right away impressed me as being competent. We had an enlightening and down to earth discussion about prostate cancer, but nothing he told me was encouraging. Then he proceeded to give me the old-fashioned finger and thumb test, referred to as a

DRE (a Digital Rectal Exam). This is a process of inserting the finger and the thumb into the rectum and actually grasping and feeling the prostate gland through a thin layer of tissue. This allows him to assess its pliability (or lack of) and to detect if the surface is smooth or rough (indicating tumors). Ideally the prostate should feel soft, smooth and symmetrical. (This is a routine process that men have endured for years any time they were subjected to physicals. Until the advent of PSA tests in the late 80s, the DRE had been about the only prostate test available. Now it is still used, but hopefully, in conjunction with PSA tests).

The doctor discovered that there was a slight enlargement of the prostate and at least two small nodules. Common sense made me realize right then that I had prostate cancer, but I wasn't in the mood to give in to it just yet. I just wanted to leave that office as quickly and politely as possible. I told him that I wasn't ready to commit myself to anything at this point, and he didn't encourage me to do so. I explained that we were scheduled for a February trip and he encouraged us to go. He indicated that there was no urgency in making a decision but that the next logical step would be a biopsy. When we left his office, I had pretty much decided that I would schedule a biopsy as soon as we returned from vacation.

Before we left for vacation, I kept an appointment I had scheduled with my cardiologist and informed him of my prostate problem. He confided that he recently went through a prostate problem that required a biopsy, which fortunately was negative. (I was comforted to learn that we were using the same urologist, whom he recommended very highly).

When we returned from vacation I contacted my urologist and scheduled a biopsy, which he would perform in his office on March 25. I reminded him that I had a mitral valve prolapse problem, which required special precaution against infection. He agreed to consult with my cardiologist about the need to use antibiotics.

I arrived for my appointment and was given an antibiotic shot in the hip an hour ahead of the biopsy process. About 30 minutes later I took six antibiotic pills, which I would continue to take for a week after the biopsy. I had been told in advance that the biopsy would be performed without anesthetics, and the pain would be no worse than getting a tooth filled. (Actually the procedure wasn't that painful). I stretched out on the operating table, lying on my side with my legs drawn up. The process was explained to me, and then it began. My rectum was greased up so instruments could be easily inserted and withdrawn. An ultrasound devise was utilized, which beamed sound waves into the body to transmit images of the prostate to a computer screen. The doctor viewed the image of the prostate on the screen to position the needle. Then he activated a control, causing the needle to insert itself into the tissue, take out a bite and withdraw. A total of six specimens were extracted, each from a different part of the prostate. The entire process took less than 15 minutes. I was told that results would be available in 7 to 10 days, so an appointment was scheduled for April 4. I had an agreement with both the nurse and the doctor that I would be called if the results became available before my appointment.

Waiting for the results of that biopsy was the most excruciating wait of my life. Apparently there are just a few labs in the country capable of evaluating biopsies. I still can't understand why a city of over 200,000 people can't manage to have its own lab, so patients wouldn't have to wait so long for test results.

On the seventh day I managed to stay close to the phone. By the eighth day, the phone scared me every time it rang. I had decided by then not to call the doctor's office: at that point, I just didn't want to know.

Finally the day of my appointment arrived, and I was driving to Dr. Callon's office. I must have been about half way there when I realized for certain that I would have bad news: both the nurse and the doctor had promised to call when they received the biopsy report, and I knew they would have called if the biopsy was negative. But they didn't!

By the time I arrived, my whole being was resonating with negative vibes. And, sure enough, when the doctor walked in, he briefly greeted me and, without waiting for a reply, he somberly confirmed my worst fears. My biopsy was positive. He said, **"you have prostate cancer."**

For a moment my mind drifted back to 1941. I am 17 years old. My Mother had been diagnosed with breast cancer and had undergone a mastectomy. Now the doctors have told her that the cancer had returned and is too far advanced to operate again. She has chosen to spend her few remaining months at home. I am the oldest of the four children still at home and the only one Dad confides in about the severity of Mother's condition. She is in pain much of the time but still insists on doing some of the many chores, even though Dad has hired a woman to help with the housework. Mother is given morphine for her pain, but gradually, as her body builds up a tolerance, the pain becomes unbearable. I am included in the nightly rotation to sit up with her as she tries to sleep in a bed we had set up for her in the living room. There are times she will drop off, but invariably she wakes up screaming with agonizing pain—and there is no way to help her. All I can do to comfort her is hold her hand and share her grief as she is dying, one night at a time.

During this period of several months, our entire family unit begins to disintegrate as Mother's control wanes. Dad's patience is increasingly stretched to the breaking point as he tries to run the household and farm at the same time. My two sisters, age 11 and 13, suffer the most, being at the age where mothers are absolutely indispensable. I am in my last year of high school and have difficulty concentrating on anything but Mother's fate. I have never considered that a time would come when she wouldn't be part of my life. Mother and I are close—we have a very special relationship. She is my best friend. Experiencing her suffering and seeing her dying torments and haunts me night and day.

I lost my Mother to cancer when she was 43 and I still bear the scars of that nightmare. When I hear the word cancer, all I think of is her excruciating pain, unfairness, hopelessness and death.

Then I was consciously back with the doctor, and he was showing me the results of my biopsy report that identified the location of cancer cells on both lobes of my prostate. In medical terms it is classified as a stage B2 (or a T2c) condition. I really didn't know what to say or what to ask. At that moment, I didn't want to talk and I wasn't in the mood for listening; I really wanted to get out of there as soon as possible. My doctor seemed uncomfortable too, but he kept talking and finally asked me to check with the secretary before leaving. She told me I was scheduled for a bone scan at Akron General Medical Center on Monday evening. This would be the next step, to determine if the cancer cells were confined to the prostate gland. I walked out to my car where I just sat, for a long time. I was experiencing the lowest point in my life and I was concerned about depressing everyone around me. Then I slowly drove home.

2

A BONE SCAN

✦

(April, 1997)

Peg accompanied me for my bone scan. We were escorted to a waiting room where I got an injection of radioactive isotope (dye) which flows and accumulates at sites of new bone formation. Because prostate cancer causes the formation of new bone, the cancer causes a "hot spot" in the scan, which will appear as a darkened area. The problem is, I found out later, that anything else that causes bone formation, such as a broken bone or arthritis, could also cause a "hot spot." It took the dye two hours to properly circulate in the body, so we used that time to go out for dinner.

The bone scan itself was a painless process which involved lying on my back, fully clothed, while the machine containing the special camera slowly moved over me, taking pictures. The technician controlled the process from her monitor. It took the machine 15 minutes to traverse the length of my body. From time to time she had me change my position in order to target pictures at a different angle. At one point, when the camera was focused on my neck area, she asked me if I had experienced any arthritis in that area. When I answered yes, she explained that this would likely account for the darker image, similar to what the existence of cancer might look like. She explained that she wasn't implying a problem, but that she just wanted more detailed pictures for the specialist who would be reading the x-ray. I did a double take when I saw my own skeleton on the monitor. It gave me an eerie feeling, like being given a premonition of the future.

When the process was completed I asked the technician how soon my doctor would have the results. She said about a week. When I questioned her further, she explained that a radiologist would read it the next day, then it would have to be written up on the proper forms and finally mailed—all of that would take about a week. This struck me as being unreasonable, and also inconsiderate. I explained that I wasn't blaming her, but that it seemed ridiculous for me to sweat out the results for a week when the doctor who reads the x-ray could easily fax the results to my doctor the next day. It was difficult for me to think that doctors and hospital administrators wouldn't be aware of the anxiety patients experience waiting for critical test results. Since my urologist was just across the street, there was no excuse for it to take a week to get there. I realized when I was voicing my frustration that I should be talking directly to the hospital administrator.

By Thursday I was on pins and needles, again. I wasn't sure I wanted a phone call. I could visualize the radiologist reading that scan and taking a closer look where he sees too much dark mass, especially down in the area of my bladder, and kidney, and liver. All it would have taken was for one little cancer cell from my prostate to have gotten into my blood stream and settled anywhere else—and all the options I might have had would have been closed. And to think, just a few months ago, my biggest worry was having rust on my Camry. Then I was jolted with the most devastating news of my life—I have prostate cancer. Just a few days later, I would feel just great if my prostate were the only place in my body that contained cancer cells.

Finally, later in the afternoon, I called my urologist's office and asked for the results of the test. They reported that it hadn't arrived but they would have it on Friday. One more day to sweat. When I returned from walking late Friday morning and saw the light blinking on my recorder I hastened to punch the button. The doctor's voice came through loud and clear, "Mr. Sandage, this is Dr. Callon calling to let you know that the scan was OK—no problem there, so you have a relaxing weekend."

3

A VISIT WITH THE RADIOLOGIST

✦

(April, 1997)

My urologist had prearranged my appointment with a radiologist for April 15. He had explained that this consultation would give me an opportunity to get any questions answered about radiation as a treatment to consider. Peg and I walked into the hospital a little early with a good deal of apprehension. After going through the inevitable paper signing process, I was turned over to a young lady who started to take me on a tour of the radiation treatment department. I hastened to explain that I wasn't there for radiation treatment, but just to talk to the doctor. But when she told me that I had 10 minutes before the doctor would be available, I might as well take the tour, in the event I should decide on radiation treatment. It was a very busy area and there seemed to be a constant flow of cancer patients coming and going. I was told that about 80 to 100 patients were receiving treatment daily in this department, which had just two radiation machines. Patients were treated each week-day for seven to eight weeks, each with his own prescribed dosage, which might change during the course of treatment. Once treatments started, they emphasized the need to avoid interruptions in the process. This caused me to wonder if patients might benefit by being treated every day, including weekends. When I later talked to a doctor about this possibility, I was told that as far as he knew, continuous treatment without weekend breaks had never been tested, and that it would be difficult to provide the necessary manpower on weekends.

After a patient completes his course of treatments, it would be six to eight more weeks before tests would be run to determine the degree of effectiveness accomplished by the radiation. I cringed at the thought of spending two months going through this repetitive daily process as well as experiencing the painful side effects radiation might cause.

Later we met with the Radiologist, Dr. Bruce, who was very informal and personable. He appeared to be in his early 40's. He made us comfortable and with his file of my medical history in front of him, got down to business. He asked me a number of pertinent questions about my medical history and made notes as I answered. He then proceeded to give me a thorough digital prostate examination, after which he started to describe his opinion of my status. He conceded that I had a serious cancer problem, which would require treatment. But the cancer was presumably localized (within the confines of the prostate) and it was in a relatively early stage. He described in detail the four or five alternatives for treatment, including two that were still experimental, and explained what each would likely accomplish and the probable side effects. He said that the type of treatment depended on the stage of the disease and the patients age and health. He further explained, "because prostate cancer cells usually spread slowly, many older men who have the disease may never need any treatment. They will likely die from some other disease before the prostate cancer would spread to vital organs. But a 65-year-old, in otherwise good health, would more likely be in jeopardy of prostate cancer catching up with him and shortening his life span—so he would be a candidate for treatment, probably surgery."

We asked a lot of questions. He gave us thoughtful and considered answers. In the final analysis, he leaned toward surgery for me, explaining "it offers the best chance of eradicating all of the cancer cells. Because you seem healthier overall and more energetic than most 72 year olds, this would be your best chance of living a full life without having cancer cut it short." He added that he felt my chances would be favorable also with radiation, but he considered surgery the only truly "golden alternative."

It was 6 PM when this session ended. We had been face to face with this specialist for two solid hours. We agreed later that we had never met a doctor before with as much wisdom and compassion, or one as forthright and deliberate in his answers. And I had certainly never before been the center of a doctor's attention for that much time.

Surgery had been my preference all along, but because of my serious heart problems, I questioned my ability to withstand the operation. I would, of course, need to consult my cardiologist and my urologist in the next few days. Before we left, I mentioned to Dr. Bruce that we had plans for a trip to Iowa and wondered if we should cancel. He pondered that question for about three seconds, and with a comforting smile said, "I've got just the remedy that's tailor-made for that problem. I'll give you prescriptions for some medication that will start shrinking those cancer tumors and will hold them in place for a few months." Then he scribbled out prescriptions for Lupron serum to be injected, as well as Casodex pills. He explained that the growth of cancer is promoted by testosterone, which is the male hormone produced by the testicles and delivered to the prostate through the blood stream. These drugs will effectively cut off the production of testosterone, robbing the cancer cells of their main source of food. We were relieved, because this "holding action" would allow us more time to make the final treatment decision.

4

AN APPOINTMENT WITH THE UROLOGIST

A day or so later I called the urologist's office to arrange an appointment to talk about my treatment preference. I informed his secretary about my conference with Dr. Bruce and his recommendation for surgery. The earliest appointment I could get was 10 days out. The next day I got a call from the urologist personally, and he was very disturbed about my apparent preference for surgery. He said that, with my heart condition, he considers surgery too high a risk. He further stated "Radiation treatment and successful surgery would have just about equal effect on my life span—so why risk the operating table." I was amazed at this call and was surprised at how strongly he questioned my ability to withstand surgery. Earlier, in his office, I remembered that he seemed to be kind of pushing me toward radiation, but also indicating he would do the surgery if I decided to go that way. We concluded by agreeing to consult with my cardiologist, who would be the best judge of whether or not my heart could withstand an operation.

I would never have anticipated that the two specialists who interviewed me and reviewed the same medical history would recommend such opposing methods of treatment. This had me in a quandary, because I respected their views and knew they were both sincere in their recommendations. But the thought of taking radiation treatments each weekday for eight weeks, and suffering the nauseating side effects, wasn't very appealing. At the same time, I wasn't in the market for taking an unnecessary risk on the operating table when there was another alternative. This waiting between appointments to keep this process going was beginning to wear on my patience.

On April 29, 1997, my wife and I arrived at the urologist's office well prepared, but not anxious, to discuss my alternatives. He informed me that he had sent a letter to my cardiologist seeking his assessment of my ability to withstand massive surgery. I reiterated that I wasn't requesting surgery, but was merely responding to the recommendation of the radiologist he had referred me to. I further stated, with probably some irritation in my voice, that I was at a high level of frustration now for the obvious reason that the two specialists I have sought out are making opposing recommendations.

He didn't challenge the opposing view, he merely restated his own, which was that, in his judgment, I wouldn't be a good risk for surgery. He explained that prostate surgery is a high-risk procedure even for a 72-year-old with a history of good health. It is a four to five hour operation, a long period for a heart patient like me to be anesthetized, subject to both blood clots and pneumonia. He again insisted that radiation would be just as effective as surgery and it would eliminate the risk of dying on the operating table.

Regardless of whether I chose surgery or radiation I was concerned about having cancer in the lymph nodes near my prostate. I stated that I had read where that seems to be the case about 30% of the time, even for patients staged as B2, as I was. He didn't dispute this statistic. Instead, he replied, "There is only one feasible way to determine if cancer has reached the lymph nodes, and that is to surgically remove some or all of them while the patient is already anesthetized and ready for surgery. Then, while the patient remains on the operating table, a pathologist would prepare a frozen section of the nodal tissue and put it under a microscope. This would add about an hour to an already lengthy surgery. If the lymph nodes were to test positive, I would, in most cases, withdraw from completing the prostate surgery and close the patient back up. Once cancer has reached the lymph nodes, it has already penetrated beyond—so an operation, or radiation for that matter, would not cure the cancer, which is the sole purpose of treatment."

This graphic disclosure was so contrary to anything I could have imagined that I just sat there in stunned disbelief. Now my alternatives had really diminished. If he had been trying to discourage me from opting for prostate surgery, he had succeeded. This was one doctor's appointment I could easily have done without. Now I had reached my greatest point of hopelessness and confusion. But I agreed to go ahead and consult with my cardiologist for whatever tests he prescribed to measure the ability of my heart to withstand an operation. It wouldn't hurt to know what kind of shape I was in.

On May 8, my cardiologist had me scheduled for a thallium stress test. I skipped breakfast and arrived at the hospital early in the morning. The tracer, a chemical that will accumulate in areas of blocked circulation, was injected into me as I went to work on the treadmill. I was hooked up to a monitor to record my pulse rate. It registered 55 as I started to walk. As the speed and elevation of the treadmill increased, I had to work harder to keep up. By the time I just about reached my limit of endurance, my pulse rate was 136 and the test was finished. I felt strong throughout and was confident that I tested well, but I wouldn't have the results for a week.

The next phase involved 15 minutes of laying on the scanning table as the images of my circulatory system were examined while my heart rate was still high. Then I had a two-hour break to allow my heart rate to return to normal, then came back for another session. It would take a week to get the results of this test, but it wouldn't really matter. I had pretty much eliminated surgery as too high a risk.

5

RESEARCHING STARTS IN EARNEST

I t had been 43 days since my biopsy and I was still going through the process of waiting for appointments and trying to educate myself about prostate cancer. I made a trip to the local American Cancer Society and asked for the appropriate information. The dozen or so pieces they provided were well written and easy to understand, but the material was dated 1987 to 1994, which made me wonder about its reliability. I encountered the same problem at the main library—no information more recent than 1994. In the last few years, I remembered reading a number of optimistic articles in newspapers about new and improved treatments for prostate cancer. I was only interested in current information. I finally resorted to the Internet and printed several dozen pages on prostate cancer entitled, "Information for Health Care Professionals," provided by the National Cancer Institute. These were reports of prostate cancer research from a large number of medical specialists and were directed to doctors and health care professionals. The material was just the detail I was looking for, and with the help of my medical dictionary, I could understand most of it. All of the information was heavily referenced, fraught with names of well-known doctors and prestigious institutions. Then my short-lived triumph was shattered. I just assumed that information from the Internet would be current, but it wasn't. The sources for each piece of information were referenced at the end. To my chagrin, the most recent date was 1994, already three years old, and the sources for the majority of the material were based on research results dating as far back as 1976. Now I began realizing that current information about prostate cancer research, from any source, was sadly lacking. Eventually I was to discover that, in recent years, although there had been a dramatic increase in the number of men encountering prostate cancer, the amount of PC research had been diminishing.

Most of this material from the Internet tracked the results of hundreds of patients who had undergone prostate cancer treatment. These patients were categorized by their staging letters (which is supposed to signify how far their cancer had advanced at the time it was detected), and by their methods of treatment. Of A and B stage patients who received radiation treatment, 50% experienced recurrence within five years. Recurrence from surgery was somewhat less, about 30%. However, the data indicated that patients undergoing surgery were younger and had less advanced cancer. I was able to digest this material and began to better understand most of the factors involved, and it was pretty scary.

In almost all of the research data I studied, the prevailing conclusion was that there is considerable under-staging by the medical profession. Many of us who are staged and treated as A's and B's are really B's & C's. A high percentage of patients are treated as though their cancer is localized in their prostate when, in fact, it has spread beyond the prostate—in which case neither radiation or surgery will stop its spread. I reread the following quote several times, "Even when the cancer appears clinically localized to the prostate gland a substantial fraction of patients will develop disseminated tumor after local therapy with surgery or irradiation. This is due to the incidence of clinical under-staging even with current diagnostic techniques. Metastatic tumor is currently not curable."

Urologists and radiologists, who review these test results regularly, must know that many patients are under-staged, and that they are providing treatment to a certain percentage of patients every year who will experience recurring cancer. In their defense, an effective and practical method to determine when cancer has spread beyond the prostate has yet to be discovered. In the meantime, based on research reports I've reviewed, they are guessing right about half of the time, and the other half of the patients are given the opportunity to be optimistic for awhile.

Later I discovered "Prostate Cancer," by Dr. Kent Wallner, published in 1996. This book would have saved me much frustration had I seen it sooner. It is easy to understand and is illustrated and organized ideally for those of us who have just discovered a prostate problem. Sadly, this book, along with some of the other material I have reviewed, confirms that if you have prostate cancer, regardless of what stage it is in, there is no consensus among medical specialists about the most effective way to treat it. Their solution is to provide the patient with a little input (far too little) and then ask him to decide which treatment he wants. At some early point I decided I would have to learn enough about it so I could make an intelligent treatment choice, and I didn't have much time. I felt overwhelmed with this responsibility. Even though I had experienced more than my share of medical problems in my life, I had never been placed in a position quite like this one where I, instead of the doctor, would make the treatment decision.

6

TREATMENT OPTIONS

Following is a synopsis of the alternatives that I reviewed and considered, and some of the "rules of thumb" along with some pitfalls.

SURGERY: only performed on men under 70 who are otherwise healthy and are staged as A or B. The risks from the operation include death associated with the anesthesia, blood clots forming in the legs or lungs and pneumonia. Other risks are the possibility of incontinence, impotency and rectal damage. In addition, the likelihood of cancer recurring is 30% in five years and 60% in ten.

EXTERNAL RADIATION: the most common treatment for men who are not eligible for surgery, but are staged A or B. Cancer cells absorb the radiation, which kills the DNA, causing the affected cells to shrink, go into remission or die.. Cancer cells are more sensitive to radiation than normal cells, however, damage to normal tissue will always occur, to varying degrees. Radiation treatments are given each week-day over a seven to eight week period. The beams of radiation are tailored by direction, intensity and duration for the individual patient. During and after treatment there are a number of possible side effects such as rectum inflammation, frequent bowl movements and urination irritation and frequency. There is also a slight risk of incontinence and a much greater likelihood of impotence (radiation damages the small blood cells which are necessary to obtain an erection). About 50% of patients with stage A or B cancer are cured or put into remission with radiation.

Cancer returns in cases where the staging assigned by the pathologist, and accepted by the urologist or the radiologist, is erroneous, and a patient, for example, is treated as a B, when in fact he is a C (he may have cancer in the lymph nodes or beyond). I emphasize this because at that point in my research, that was my greatest concern (I was staged as a B).

IMPLANT RADIATION: the direct placement of radioactive pellets into the prostate. Patients are usually limited to men under 70 with reasonably small prostates and staged A or B (cancer localized in the prostate). They would also need to be in generally good health otherwise. General side effects are less severe than with external radiation except for urination, which is more frequent and causes a burning sensation. The likelihood of a cure is similar to surgery. The minor surgery takes about an hour and requires about one or two days in the hospital. My interest in this treatment was restrained only because long-term results were not yet available, but short-term results were encouraging.

CRYOTHERAPY: this is a process of freezing the cancer cells and is too new for me to consider. This treatment was being increasingly used for salvage (recurring) cancer treatment, but substantial side effects had been reported and what little information about results that was available, wasn't considered reliable.

HORMONAL THERAPY: prostate cancer is partially dependent on the presence of male hormones for its growth. Therefore, drugs used to deplete male hormones will cause most prostate cancers to go into remission, There is very little agreement among doctors about when to use this treatment. It is known that continuous usage will encourage the surviving tumor cells to develop resistance to hormonal therapy. Right from the beginning, I started taking a hormonal drug (Casodex) to hold my cancer in remission for a few months while deciding what to do.

ORCHIECTOMY (castration): since the testicles produce nearly all the male hormones, this is an effective way to deplete male hormone production. Most patients have a built-in male psyche against even discussing such a drastic step—at least in the early stages. I didn't consider it.

PITUITARY INTERFERENCE: the pituitary gland, located on the underside of the brain, releases a hormone that circulates through the blood and signals the testicles to produce testosterone. This gland is another point where a hormonal drug can be targeted to further limit the production of testosterone. For this purpose, I was taking Lupron injections, again in an effort to hold my cancer in remission temporarily. Unfortunately, this treatment alone is not effective long range.

Those are the treatment alternatives I had reviewed and studied, but I wasn't enamored with any of them. There were a number of elements involved in my research, which bothered me a great deal. In both the written material I had studied as well as several consultations with medical specialists, the subject of "life expectancy" was a dominant factor. It isn't that I hadn't thought about death before. I was in combat in World War II and on a number of occasions, with artillery and mortar shells indiscriminately raining down on us, I actually anticipated death, as did we all. But there we had no choices to make—death was determined pretty much by the luck of the draw—and we knew and accepted that. But this was my first experience at talking about death so openly and playing such a key role in making decisions that might well establish when it occurs. The determination of which treatment would be best for me went something like this. At 72 years old, let's say the actuaries would give me 12 more years without this cancer. Now the question becomes, will the cancer get me before I die from something else. That type of reasoning, along with using "averages" to assess how long patients using treatment A lived compared to those who chose treatment B, is a real turnoff. Who is average?

7

THE STAGING PROCESS

One of the most critical concerns I had, as I learned more and more about prostate cancer, is the process of assigning each patient a staging number. Staging is merely numbers that represent the medical professionals' best estimate of the tumor's maturity and progress (how much is present and how far it has advanced). The first "staging" is the PSA test number that, in my case, was 10. This got me an immediate appointment with my urologist, and a biopsy. The next "staging" is performed by the pathologist. In the process of rendering his biopsy report, he provides a "Gleason Score." This score probably carries more weight than any other does because it is the only test result that comes from actually looking at the cancer cells through a microscope. The pathologist attempts to determine the "aggression level" of the tumor by comparing the shape and configuration of the cancer cells to that of normal cells. Apparently, the greater the differentiation, the greater is the aggression level. This process is obviously somewhat subjective, as two pathologists might score them differently. The scores range from 2 to 10, with 10 being the most aggressive. My Gleason score was 5.

And finally, the urologist, after considering all the evidence available, and leaning heavily on the report from the pathologist, renders his "staging" score. This score is particularly crucial because it influences which treatment remedies will be appropriate. The scores range from A to D, with numbered subdivisions associated with each letter, to more precisely define the cancer's status. A, for example, is the least serious letter, and indicates a tumor involving less than 5% of tissue resected. A B1 would indicate tumors in one lobe of the prostate—a

B2 (such as mine) indicates tumors in both lobes but presumably localized in the prostate. C and D staging would indicate that the tumor has spread beyond the confines of the prostate, which would then greatly restrict treatment options.

Research reports are generally in agreement about the probability of recurrence of cancer after radiation treatment. For instance, 30 to 50% of staged A and B patients will have recurrence within five years, as will 60 to 75% of staged C. Statistics based on Gleason scores show that those with scores of 2 to 6 will have a 25% chance of recurrence in five years and a 57% recurrence with scores of 7 to 10. Test results also show a close correlation between PSA test results and Gleason scores. In other words, the higher the PSA, the more likely the Gleason score will be high as well.

The recurrence of cancer after surgery is a little less pessimistic than after radiation, but that may be because surgery is usually not performed if staging scores are high. Even so, there is still a significantly high recurrence rate with surgery, and an even higher rate of debilitating side effects. Granted that the research material I studied is several years old, because newer material is not available, I'm doubtful that more recent research will show improved statistics. *There is consensus among just about all the research specialists that under-staging is prevalent among doctors, probably because they want to hold out hope when confronting their patients.* In addition, it is almost impossible to accurately determine the status of cancer, especially in the early stages—even with biopsies. For one thing, from a practical standpoint, tissue for biopsies can only be extracted from one side of the prostate, which leaves a sizable portion of it unexamined. And even the tissue that is removed from one side, which is usually six samples, constitutes a very small percentage of even that portion of the prostate. Granted that if cancer is detected in any of the samples, that patient does have cancer of the prostate. But if all of the tissue samples which are removed test negative, that patient may still have cancer but the needles missed it. An example of this is the famous golfer, Arnold Palmer. When he was suspected of having PC, he was put through 17 biopsies before finally getting a positive reading. Obviously, he had cancer during that entire period.

8

RUNNING OUT OF TIME

✦

(MAY 1997)

The biggest turn off I experienced was from a visit with a well-meaning friend. After learning that I had prostate cancer, he said, "It certainly is unfortunate to have cancer of any kind. But, if you have to have cancer, prostate cancer is the best one to have because the medical profession has made so many great advances in dealing with it in recent years." And to think, up to a few months before, I may have made the same statement. It is now becoming increasingly obvious to me that in the area of understanding and effectively treating and curing prostate cancer, progress has been moving at a snail's pace for at least a half a century. In contrast to what my acquaintances and the general public think, enough advances are just not coming on stream. Hopefully, there are advances currently in the research stage, but with the exception of the PSA test, which is very significant, basic treatment has changed very little in the last 25 years. And as long as most people continue to be unaware of the lack of progress, there will be no public outcry, and real advances are likely to be slow in coming (something to do with the squeaky wheel syndrome).

As I realized that it had been 66 days since my biopsy, I became increasingly concerned about making a final treatment decision. When I got my telephone call from my cardiologist, I learned that my stress test was favorable. He would still require me to undergo a catheterization in order to evaluate the status of my circulatory system before he would approve surgery. However, I had just about eliminated that alternative anyway, but it was comforting to realize that my daily fast walks had strengthened my heart muscles. Within a few days I would be talking to my radiologist to get some final questions answered. It was my intention to start whatever treatment I would decide on as soon as we returned from a trip to Iowa.

Dr. Bruce called the day before our appointment and canceled, but he agreed to a telephone conference later that evening. When he called back, I informed him that I was leaning toward having my lymph nodes removed and biopsied and then start radiation treatment if they should test negative. When I asked for his reaction, he said that this would have merit and agreed to touch base with Dr. Callon, who would be doing that surgery. I voiced my frustration about the amount of time being consumed waiting for appointments with doctors and my desire to minimize further delays. He consoled me by reminding me that we actually weren't delaying because I was already being treated with hormones. We scheduled a meeting for May 30, which would be soon after our return from Iowa, at which time I planned to have made my treatment decision.

At that point, I was more concerned about whether or not cancer had already spread to my lymph nodes. I didn't want to go through the torture of a whole sequence of radiation treatments, then learn that it accomplished nothing. At the same time, I wasn't sure I really wanted to know if I had cancer in my lymph nodes either. Based on my research, the odds were about 70 to 30 in my favor—but I was still in my pessimistic mode.

My sister had mailed me a number of books and papers on a variety of nontraditional treatments for cancer. This material promoted rigid dieting and exercise, and taking vitamins and supplements. The theory was that as you age, your immune system becomes less efficient and certain natural foods and mineral supplements can help reinforce it and increase its ability to ward off diseases and sickness. This theory made a lot of sense and I would intend to further research nutritional alternatives. But with my prostate cancer at such a critical stage, I wasn't about to turn my back on the medical profession and rely solely on alternative treatments.

9

DECISION TIME

❖

(May, 1997)

We returned from vacation, and two days before my scheduled appointment with Dr. Bruce, I attended my first support group meeting. This group, sponsored by the American Cancer Society, is limited to prostate cancer victims, and is named "Man to Man." The speaker was Dr. Eric Klein, who is head of the section of Urologic Oncology at the Cleveland Clinic Foundation's Department of Urology. He had a very impressive resume and I not only gave him my full attention, but I asked questions and managed to maneuver some private dialog with him afterward. When I advised him of my age, my health limitations, my PSA grade and my staging number, he not only recommended radiation, but he endorsed both my urologist and my radiologist as being experienced and competent. His final statement was, "in my opinion; I would definitely recommend radiation. And with your cancer at such an early stage, you should feel confident that radiation would handle it." This short visit did a lot for my morale. During the next two days I began to feel more optimistic about my probability of being a genuine B2 patient, with no cancer in my lymph nodes.

When Peg and I met with Dr. Bruce, as scheduled, I informed him that I was backing away from having my lymph nodes surgically removed, as I had indicated in my last telephone conference. Instead, I was now willing to proceed with the assumption that my cancer hadn't spread beyond the prostate, which my staging numbers would suggest. He agreed that the chances were strong in my favor. We had a lengthy discussion about the equipment used at AGMC compared to Cleveland Clinic. Cleveland used a newer, more sophisticated radiation machine, which allowed them to apply slightly higher doses of radiation and to apply it with a bit more precision. Dr. Cross explained that the more updated equipment was too new to have been proven to be better. He also indicated that he applies somewhat higher radiation doses than the textbook prescribes. I saw this as a plus. As we talked, I was comparing the advantage of newer equipment in Cleveland, which would require driving almost 100 miles a day for treatment, versus older equipment that was tried and proven and was 15 minutes from home. I also was convinced that I would have especially good access to Dr. Bruce, which I must refrain from abusing, and he had already exhibited genuine concern and candor. Plus, he was a good listener. Throughout this visit, at the same time I was weighing and evaluating responses to my questions, I was focusing on the magnitude of the life or death decision I was about to make. The unfortunate fact was that if radiation was applied to my prostate, and it failed—I wouldn't get a second chance. Radiation treatment modifies the molecular structure of cells in such a way that it can't be effectively applied the second time.

The time had arrived. I decided to make my decision now. I still wasn't completely satisfied, but my decision-making time had expired. I asked Dr. Bruce to take over the responsibility of my radiation treatment process, and he agreed to do so as soon as it could be scheduled.

Although I had been on a hormonal treatment program for the past two months, it had been four months since my blood was drawn, which led to the diagnosis of cancer. Then we had taken a pre-planned trip to Florida and another one to Iowa. During and in between these trips I had researched and studied and learned a great deal about prostate cancer. I had worked my way through each of the conventional and then the unconventional treatment alternatives, evaluating and considering, getting a second opinion, and asking questions. My choice was reached purely by eliminating one conventional treatment that I didn't qualify for, and because I chickened out of selecting a promising non-conventional treatment that was too new. Hopefully, those who come later will have better options.

During these trying days I have lived the various predictable stages of being a cancer victim—denial, disbelief, betrayal and anger—lots of anger. Anger at myself initially, and guilt, for not having acted sooner—especially as I appreciate more and more the life saving value of early detection. Anger at the medical profession for not being able to tell me, convincingly, that they can provide a totally satisfactory solution. Anger at their snail-paced progress, and yes, the lack of their effort to demand more funding to intensify prostate cancer research. Anger that the medical profession, all these years, has adamantly refrained from even investigating the potential merits of "unconventional" treatment alternatives—right where amazing benefits may be lurking. Anger that while the medical profession is certainly aware of its ineffectiveness in dealing with prostate cancer, it condones, and may even contribute, to the general public's unfounded opinion of its success. And anger that it was necessary for me, a medical neophyte, to attempt my own medical research in order to make an informed treatment decision.

After completing this research process and making my treatment choice, which turned out to be the one that my urologist had suggested originally, I accepted the fact that it was the best I could do at that time. However, I didn't intend to rely on radiation alone. I had already started studying how the body works, and the role that different foods and supplements can play in fortifying the body to combat cancer. I had been cautioned by my radiologist that taking supplements would conflict with the hormonal treatment I was on and the radiation treatment that I would be starting. Both of these treatments were in direct conflict with nutritional supplements; hormones and radiation attempt to kill cells, while nutritional supplements attempt to fortify them.

Ironically, for awhile, I would be fighting in concert with the "cell killers" instead of the cell fortifiers.

10

RADIATION TREATMENT PRELIMINARIES

⟐

(June, 1997)

O n June 10 Dr. Bruce started the process of determining exactly where to apply the radiation beams. I was given a computerized tomography (a CT or Cat Scan) of my pelvic area. This machine used a rotating x-ray beam to take a series of pictures from a variety of angles. A computer processes this information and produces three-dimensional images of my prostate and surrounding bones, organs and tissue.

Two days later I was permitted to review this Cat Scan with Dr. Bruce and I felt a little queasy seeing my own prostate and surrounding organs lit up on the screen. Some of the images were crisscrossed with lines, 16 to the inch, forming a grid. This Scan provided evidence of where the contamination was concentrated, which Dr. Bruce had highlighted with a marking pencil. He showed me that my prostate was relatively small, which was a plus. He said that the cancer was concentrated in such a way that he wouldn't need to treat a very large area of the surrounding tissue. As a result, I would likely suffer only minor side effects. This session was a welcome morale booster, and it had a calming affect.

The next phase of the treatment planning process involved laying on my back on a special higher-powered x-ray machine called a "Simulator." The therapist's mission now was to follow the prescription of Dr.

Bruce and delineate, on my pelvis, the points through which the radiation beams should be directed in order to reach the internal target. Measurements were taken and marks were drawn on my pelvis. It was obvious that this was a very critical process by the numerous times my body was moved and marks were changed. Finally I was asked to lie very still in the position they had determined I would assume for the treatments, and the x-ray was taken. The therapist took the x-ray into another room so Dr. Bruce could evaluate its accuracy. This process was repeated several times, with x-rays being taken from my front and rear, as well as from each side.

I learned later that the process Dr. Bruce so meticulously uses to determine the radiation beam's point of entry involves applying both the CAT Scan image, as well as the x-ray, to a grid. This process allows measurements to be taken from certain bone structures, which are common to both the CAT Scan and the x-ray, thereby allowing corresponding measurements to be taken from my actual bone structure. This is a very important and exacting procedure which is done not only initially but is rechecked periodically during the course of treatment. And of course, it is done again as the target area is changed.

Once these critical points were determined and verified, permanent pinhead-sized tattoos were applied at these strategic locations on my pelvis and to each hip. Some of these tattoos identified where the radiation beam was to be aimed in order to hit the prescribed target. Others were positioned as markers for sidewall and ceiling mounted laser beams to target in on to ensure that my body was in exactly the same position each day.

Then my "simulation" was completed and I was prepped to start treatments. The therapist advised me that I had just two choices for treatment time—6:40 AM or 5:30 PM. I looked at him, expecting him to start laughing, but he wasn't joking. I opted for the early morning.

On Sunday night, I set the alarm for 5:45 AM and then tossed and turned all night. I surely was apprehensive about starting treatment, but I was also having hot flashes from my hormone treatment, which had added to my discomfort ever since I started taking it. Peg insisted on accompanying me for treatments, just as she had on most of my medical trips. I got up Monday morning, did my normal chores and put on athletic pants and a pullover shirt. We were at the hospital 10 minutes ahead of time. The therapist came in to get me and, announced that my first treatment was postponed till the next day. Then she proceeded to put me through the simulation process again, apparently as another precautionary measure to verify that the markings were accurately placed to line up with the radiation target areas. This extra display of caution did a lot to raise my comfort level, and nudged me one notch closer to a feeling of confidence in Dr. Bruce. The trip the next day would be for real.

11

RADIATION STARTS FOR REAL

Tomorrow came, and it was June 17, 1997, the real day of my first radiation treatment. We were early as usual. This time, Ron, the male therapist, escorted me to a different room and I took my position on the table of the "linear accelerator" for the first time—the machine that would be used to apply the radiation treatments. He explained that my radiation treatment would be given from the side every other day and then from front and rear on alternate days. By using this technique, damage to the normal tissue, between the surface and the infected target area, would be spared every other day, while the target area itself would be "zapped" every day. This method would allow the good tissue a better chance to recover. I learned that the initial radiation treatment target area measured 11.5 x 8.5 centimeters (about the size of my billfold).

Ron proceeded to position my body so that the laser beams from each side wall would hit the tattoo marks on my hips, and the red beam from the ceiling would line up with the tattoo in the center of my pelvis, thereby confirming that my body was properly positioned for the prescribed treatment. At this point he pushed a button to rotate the gantry (a large arm that holds the beaming devise) 90 degrees clockwise, to line up with the tattoo on my right hip. He let me know that we were all set and that now he would, in old military terms, be firing for effect. He then left the room where he could control the machine and at the same time observe me through a window. I learned that this procedure is required to protect the technicians from over exposure to radiation. They also wear a device that will change color to warn them if the radiation accumulation level is too high.

In a few seconds I heard the clicking noise of the radiation being shot through my body—I felt nothing. I started counting the seconds and got to 26 before it stopped. Then Ron came back in, re-verified my position, adjusted the machine arm 180 degrees to the other hip, and left. The clicking started again, and this time, in my mind's eye, I saw the normal cells in my prostate getting zapped, along with the cancer cells that were feeding on them. It flashed through my mind that only two times in my life had I given up part of my body: some skin from my penis when I was circumcised as an infant, and my tonsils when I was about eight—neither given up voluntarily. As the clicking continued, I started visualizing those poisonous beams going through my skin, my muscle, my soft tissue and into my prostate gland, and right on through the live flesh on the other side—damaging and savaging everything in its path on its 26 second mission. The most eerie, helpless feeling enveloped me. It was as if my body was being invaded and would never be the same again—like I would imagine a woman might feel as she is being raped. Then the clicking stopped. Physically, I felt nothing. It was painless. Emotionally it will take some getting used to.

Successive treatments were uneventful. Each morning we returned home, ate breakfast and headed to the mall for our daily 30-minute walk. I was spending several hours a day reviewing books and whatever I could pull off the Internet concerning prostate cancer. I learned that the angle radiation beams are directed vary, depending on factors such as the shortest distance to the target, what vital organs can be missed by changing the angle etc. In my case, the treatments, from each of the four directions, were beamed at 90 degrees. The diameter of a beam of radiation is at its smallest when it enters the body, and enlarges as it progresses to the target, similarly to water coming out of a hose. Adversely, the intensity, or strength, of the beam of radiation intensifies as it goes deeper into the body. This is an advantage in that it allows the tissue nearer the surface to heal faster. I'm beginning to appreciate the essence of a statement I had read recently, that it is not difficult to kill cancer with radiation when it can be applied directly to the tumors—the problem is in getting it through the tissue and vital organs without destroying the good stuff, and still get sufficient radiation to the cancer to destroy it. It does no good to cure the cancer and kill the patient. Another book I read states that the ideal result of radiation therapy is achieved when the tumor is completely eradicated and the surrounding normal tissues show minimal evidence of structural or functional injury. It further states that this result is seldom achieved—and that the practical result is to minimize damage to normal cells, and that different normal cells have varying tolerances for radiation. The more I learn about the process of using radiation to treat prostate cancer, the more difficult it is to accept the fact that, with all of its limitations and repercussions, we haven't discovered a less archaic alternative.

Each Monday I was scheduled for a conference with my radiologist, which I would take full advantage of by having my questions written out in advance. I wanted to understand radiation therapy more thoroughly by the time I was finished with treatments. At the first conference I asked the doctor if I should continue hormonal treatment, which I had been on for 60 days. He said I could stop it if I wanted to, but that in his opinion, within a few years, research would show that patients would benefit from hormonal treatment two months before and two months after radiation. He further explained that hormonal treatment kills off some of the cancer cells and shrinks the prostate, which lessens the workload for the radiation treatment. A smaller target will usually result in less radiation damage to the bladder and rectum. I decided to gain this advantage and put up with the annoying hot flashes a little longer.

I thought he was pulling my leg when he asked me to try to come to treatments each morning with a full bladder. But he was serious, explaining that this would help maintain a consistency in the position of the prostate gland in relation to the bladder, minimizing bladder damage. Heading for the pot the first thing each morning would be a difficult habit to change.

Another question I asked, which I had been pondering since my previous brief discussion, got a surprising response. I wondered if patients might do better if they were given radiation treatments seven days a week instead of five. I explained my concern about backsliding on weekends. I explained that I was keenly aware of how skipping a few days from exercise will take a toll. His reply was that they might backslide some, but there is no way to know for sure at this time. First, he would have a hard time getting people to work on weekends. Second, all the research, which has become the basis for how to apply the treatment, such as dosage, strength and duration, as well as all other aspects of application, had been based on a five day work week. These facts alone would negate an ability to change to a seven day a week treatment program for years to come. I was amazed at that response, but that was realism in the medical world I guess. I appreciated his candor.

Now I had completed 13 treatments and had yet to feel any side effects from radiation, but I expected to feel its effects any time now. I had just enjoyed a 4th of July three-day weekend and hoped that "time off" hadn't resulted in any backsliding. Based on 35 to 40 treatments scheduled, I was about a third of the way through already and had actually kind of taken to such an early morning routine: I got a chance to see the sun rise, we could walk when it was still cool, and by the time we finished breakfast we had most of the morning to do other things.

I was 50 years old in 1975 when I had open-heart surgery. This caused a rather dramatic change in our life style, especially our eating habits. We practically eliminated red meat, along with French fries and most other high fat foods. We switched to skim milk, whole wheat bread, eliminated sugar and salt and ate more raw fruits and vegetables. I also started taking vitamin C and E, along with lecithin and bran.

Then, in 1983, when I had a heart attack, I started a daily fast-walking program, which I have maintained, and I intensified even further my program of eating healthy food. So it was distressing to learn that during treatments, I was to follow certain dietary restrictions to minimize the intestinal cramping and diarrhea that radiation usually causes. And these restrictions required that I basically take roughage out of my diet for the duration. I was to eat white bread for the first time in 22 years, and discontinue eating foods with high fiber content such as raw fruit and vegetables. I tried to eat decent quantities of food even though I wasn't enjoying it as much. During treatment, I was weighed weekly, and noticed a slight drop in weight each time. I started looking forward to getting back to eating healthy food again.

Since I started treatments, I was trying to be alert to everything that was happening so I could report it accurately. The problem was that I couldn't see anything but the ceiling during a treatment because I was immobilized on my back and was cautioned not to even move my head. So, on the weekly sessions with Dr. Bruce, I planned to get some of the technical questions answered so I could better understand what was happening. Right after the 19th treatment, as I started asking the doctor questions about protons and target dimensions etc., he politely requested that I limit my questions solely to any immediate problems I was experiencing with the treatments. He explained that because his time was very restricted, this was the only way he could maintain his responsibilities to the other patients. He also asked me to discontinue questioning his therapists, which I had done occasionally. This unexpected reprimand naturally upset me, although I appreciated and understood his position. It was just that I knew from experience that if I didn't grasp the technical aspects of each step along the way, my narration of it would suffer. However, he did offer to give me an hour of his time several weeks out, which actually was pretty generous of a very busy doctor.

On July 16 I kept a routine appointment with my family physician, who I will call Dr. Stevens. Ever since I took the initiative to get a PSA test, and then discovered that I had cancer, I had blamed my doctor for not having scheduled me for regular yearly tests (which certainly would have discovered it sooner). So I hadn't been looking forward to this appointment. I had made a point to have him copied on all my tests relating to prostate cancer, so I assumed that he wouldn't be anxious to see me either. And sure enough, when he came into the office, it was obviously an uncomfortable moment for us both. But I was determined to have a conversation about what was bugging me. This was particularly difficult for me because Dr. Stevens is an especially nice guy, and we had always enjoyed a good relationship. He was sitting there seemingly kind of waiting for me to break the ice. So I started it off with, "have you received all the test results to bring you up to date with what I'm going through with my prostate cancer problem?" He nodded yes and started looking through my file that he had on his lap. I continued "my file would show that my PSA tested 4.8 in 1994, and I remember that you referred to it as being a 'high normal.' So didn't you think that scheduling another test in 1995, or even in 1996 surely would have been in order?"

He didn't say anything, but he looked up and slowly shook his head yes. Then I just couldn't restrain from saying, "A PSA test in 1995 might very well have discovered cancer enough earlier to make a substantial difference in my life span." At that point he made some reference to PSA tests not always being valid, and my instantaneous reply was that mine certainly was. I knew in advance that criticizing him would be uncomfortable, but I had carried some bitterness around so long, I just had to let it out. And in addition, I truly felt that he deserved to hear what I told him, for his own enlightenment. So I guess maybe something was accomplished—I vented my frustration and he may put more weight on PSA tests.

Dr. Stevens is not only very personable, but he is a very progressive doctor. He had been extremely beneficial to me in the area of my cardiovascular problems, and he seemed to always be a year or two ahead of the pack in dispensing new medical advice. So his apparent resistance to advocating, or even accepting, PSA tests really astounded me, because at this time it is, without question, the very best test available to detect prostate cancer. I had read that there were still a large number of doctors who had used the digital rectal exam for years and felt they had a special talent for being able to diagnose prostate problems that way. In such cases, they apparently felt they were doing justice to their patient by ignoring PSA—when in fact, these two tests surely should be used in tandem. Before I went into this session, I confided to a friend that if Dr. Stevens didn't share some blame for not having scheduled a follow-up PSA test, I would change doctors. I was satisfied that, although he didn't verbalize much, his demeanor reflected some remorse.

12

PROBLEMS ALONG THE WAY

The same day I took my 22nd treatment, I was also scheduled for my final Lupron (hormone) injection. I remembered that when I took my second shot, the nurse had failed to record which hip she injected. So when I went for my third shot, with no record to guide her, she guessed wrong and injected the same hip as before. Consequently, I had a very painful hip for about three days. I discovered that their written policy required them to alternate hips to avoid the kind of pain I endured. This time, when she told me that once again the nurse had made no record, I decided to give them a hard time. I politely refused to allow her to inject me. This created a little excitement in the department until another nurse referred to a computer report that did identify which hip was last injected. As a result of my stubbornness, she injected the proper hip and I experienced very little pain. I trust the discipline improved in that department and maybe I did a favor for future patients.

On my first day of radiation treatment I had sat in the waiting room next to another patient, Harold Witner. During the course of my treatments we had the opportunity to visit for a few minutes every morning, so we gradually became well acquainted. He had been in the navy during WW II. Afterwards he married Ruby (his high school sweetheart), went to work for Goodyear and had been retired for the past ten years. Harold had bought his wife a pair of dogs two years earlier as she was recovering from a bout with her second stroke. I met and visited with her on one of the occasional times she accompanied Harold to the hospital. He was receiving treatment for cancer of the throat, as well as for one side of his face. His face and neck were very red and sore, even though he was using a salve, which apparently didn't provide much relief. Just a few days later, when I arrived at the waiting room, Harold was more distraught than usual. He told me that Ruby had suffered a mild heart attack the prior night and was rushed to Barberton Hospital. He was thoroughly beat from lack of sleep. The next morning I was greeted with the news that Ruby had been moved to AGMC and that during the night she suffered another heart attack, a severe one. The following day she received a catherization, and a day or two later she had undergone a triple by-pass operation. When she came out of surgery she developed a rapid heartbeat condition, which they had difficulty stopping. And in addition, she had water in her lungs, which, if not remedied, would likely cause pneumonia. Then, on top of all that, he told me that their two dogs were so rambunctious that, in his condition, he didn't think he could continue to handle them and was thinking of having them put away. These were beautiful dogs that cost a thousand dollars, and Ruby was crazy about them. And to think that, before I encountered Harold, I thought I had problems.

About a week in advance, I was informed that I was going to be put through another "simulation process," which would reduce the target area of my radiation. On July 21 I went through this process. This time a regular black felt tip marker was used, instead of tattoos, to mark up my hips and pelvic areas. This eliminated any confusion with the permanent tattoo marks in correctly positioning by body each time. A few days later I met with my radiologist. He explained that the original target not only included the prostate, but the seminal vesicles surrounding the prostate as well. Based on all the test results he had reviewed, plus his own gut feel, he didn't think the cancer had moved beyond the prostate. So in order to get the greatest advantage from the remaining treatments, he was restricting the target area to just the prostate. I relished this change because I saw it as a positive.

13

SOME RADIATION HISTORY

During my treatments, I had continued to study everything I could find to better understand prostate cancer—all elements of it. I thought I had hit the jackpot when I learned that the hospital had a library assessable to patients. However, when I investigated, I was disappointed to discover that the library was just a small computer room with a librarian available to help medical staff and patients extract information from the Internet. Although the librarian was most cooperative, and printed some semi-useful material, I couldn't seem to get the kind of technical information I wanted. Finally I was referred to the Northeastern Ohio University College Of Medicine, just 22 miles away. This was just what I was looking for and I spent many productive hours scanning and copying applicable portions of their textbooks.

The use of radiation for human therapy purposes had its origin in Paris in the 1920s. Researchers experimented by irradiating the testes of rams with x-rays. It was soon learned that it was impossible to sterilize the animal with a single dose without causing a severe reaction to the skin of the scrotum. Further testing proved that if the dosage was reduced in intensity (fractionated), and applied over a period of time, sterilization was achieved with only minor skin damage. The success of this test soon led to starting similar experiments on human beings. After much experimenting, applicators that would provide consistent and controllable dose rates were developed. The next requirement was to make these machines non-radioactive, to protect the hospital therapists. Even though this was accomplished, therapists today all wear warning devices, which change color if too much radiation is present. Through the '30s and '40s, technical advances were made in the ability to produce much higher energy generators, which increasingly proved advantageous. In the 1950s, the first generation of medical linear accelerators was invented and became a mainstay in all large hospitals. The machine that was used on me was a Varian model 1800 linear accelerator (1800 MEV energy capacity) a direct descendant of the original, but more powerful and more sophisticated.

Over half of all patients with cancer will, at some point in the course of their treatment, receive radiation therapy. This is particularly true with prostate cancer. Any tumor can be cured with enough radiation. The limiting factor involved in its application is the tolerance limits of the body's normal tissues, which the radiation beams, must go through to deliver its energy to the tumor. Therefore, it is extremely critical that treatment planning and application be executed very precisely and with great care. There is no value in curing the tumor and killing the patient. Unfortunately, normal cells are as sensitive to radiation as are tumors, but radiation normally has to invade normal cells to reach tumors. Fortunately, normal cells have a slight advantage in their ability to recover from damage, and in addition, tumors have more cells in a sensitive phase of growth, which adds to their vulnerability to destruction by radiation. And, depending on the condition of the immune system, normal cells have the ability to regenerate and divide to recover from adversity. Larger tumors, which are often present when cancer is not detected early, are more resistant to radiation. In these cases, the amount of energy necessary to destroy the tumors may require more radiation than the body can withstand without serious injury. One of the more recent ways of dealing with this was to apply hormonal treatment in advance of applying radiation. Hormones will attack the testosterone, which is the primary source of food which cancer cells require for growing and multiplying. By depriving them, they will shrink, and in the process, become more potent victims for radiation. This was the course of action that my doctor was applying to me, but it apparently had not yet been universally applied—probably because its value had yet to be thoroughly evaluated over time. I later learned that continuous hormonal treatment will encourage the development of resistance to hormonal therapy in the surviving tumor cells. Every treatment seems to have its limitations.

14

TREATMENT EXTENDED

✦

(July 1997)

When I walked into the waiting room on Monday, July 28, and saw the downcast expression on Harold's face, I knew before he told me—Ruby had died on Sunday. They had finally subdued her rapid heartbeat and sent her home Sunday morning. Harold said that she was anxious to get home but she wasn't very talkative and it was obvious that she wasn't feeling well. That evening, about bedtime, she shrugged off his offer to help her go to the bathroom. After awhile he went in to check on her and she told him to call the paramedics, which he did. She died of another heart attack before they reached the hospital. Having had two strokes, plus the worry about Harold's problem, and then two heart attacks, it was just too much for that 75 year old woman. And sending her home just one day after being in intensive care probably wasn't very helpful either. Harold was very depressed and told me that he might discontinue taking any more treatments, especially the chemotherapy that was scheduled after he finished radiation.

My doctor notified me that he was increasing my number of treatments from 35 to 38. Since the original larger target area had already received 25 treatments, the balance, 13 more treatments, would be directed exclusively to the prostate. I had read in one of the medical journals that sometimes, if a radiation patient doesn't suffer many side effects, it might be because the doctor is a little overly cautious in the strength or the duration of the treatments. I had already determined that I would rather have too many than too few—knowing that once the treatments conclude, I could never have them again. So I was pleased to get the additional three, which meant that I had just two more weeks to go. I verified that I could then return to my normal diet. It would be a relief to get back to eating healthy food.

When I arrived for treatment number 30 on Tuesday morning, two days after Ruby died, Harold was in a surprisingly relaxed and optimistic mood. He explained that he had completed all the arrangements, including a graveside service to be conducted the next day. They had no children or relatives, except for one distant cousin. He confided that he had decided to go ahead with all of his treatments that on the prior day he was going to discontinue. His eyes lit up when he told me that the ship he served on during W.W.II was holding a reunion in San Diego in September, and he was thinking of going. He'd passed up prior invitations because his wife never wanted to go. He would go this time if he got enough of his strength back.

Even before I started my radiation treatments, I had gleaned some important information about the process from medical books. I knew how crucial it was to reposition the body precisely on the marks each time, because if the beam of radiation enters the surface of the body even a few centimeters off the mark, by the time its energy reaches the target area, it would be an inflated number of centimeters off, thereby lessening its effectiveness. The therapists who perform the treatments were required to have had a minimum of two years of x-ray training and another year to qualify to perform radiation. During the course of my treatments, I had the services of at least five different therapists, and I noticed that all of them, with the exception of one individual, were very methodical and took considerable time to line up my body just right. Therefore I was uncomfortable when the "speedy" therapist came in, afraid that he wasn't as precise as the others were. At one point I thought of mentioning it to the doctor, then I changed my mind. It reminded me of where I had been getting my hair cut for the last 25 years. There is one barber there who invariably cuts my hair twice as fast as any of the others, but I could never find any fault with the result. In fact, he may give the best haircut. It might be, in the radiation treatment room, that all the therapists are equally effective—I'm not sure. But, because I knew how critical it was to hit the mark each time, I was more comfortable with those who took more time.

15

MY SUPPORT GROUP EXPERIENCE

A t a location near me, a prostate cancer support group, sponsored by the National Cancer Society, meets monthly. The first two meetings I attended had appropriate speakers who provided very helpful information and they remained until all of our questions were answered. At my third meeting a speaker wasn't scheduled and our facilitator led the group in open discussion. There were five or six of the seemingly older men, including the facilitator, who dominated the discussion. It soon becomes apparent that some of these men were living with serious surgery or radiation treatment side effects, such as impotence or incontinence—or both. There were few remedies suggested to reduce the frequent nightly trips to the bathroom. One man commented on his moderate success at getting and sustaining an erection by using a recently available device. Another shared his experience at trying a number of devices that didn't help and finally decided, "to hell with it—it just wasn't worth it for either my wife or me." Others compared the side effects of a variety of hormone drugs they had used, including one that was effective for 90 days.

As this discussion continued, it struck me that the initial treatment each of these men had experienced three, four, or six years ago, had failed. At the time prostate cancer was originally diagnosed, based on their comments, they each had chosen either external radiation or surgery. And in each of these cases a likely scenario was that there was a flaw of some kind in the medical diagnosis or application of treatment.

In the case of those who had surgery, either cancer had already spread beyond the tissue that was removed or the surgeon may have been overly cautious when removing tissue near vital areas in his attempt to avoid causing incontinence or impotence—and this remaining tissue may have contained some cancer cells. In the case of those who had radiation treatments, the pathologist may have under-staged them. For example, turning in a report to the urologist with a rating that would indicate the likelihood that cancer was "localized" in the prostate when in fact it had already spread. Knowing this would have ruled out radiation as a remedy. Or one of a number of miscalculations or errors could have occurred in applying the radiation, allowing some cancer cells to survive. The reality was that whatever was done didn't work—at least for these men. When I realized that I had probably evaluated their situations accurately, I was very uncomfortable and depressed.

The way the facilitator of that session used the last five minutes to wind down the meeting really amazed me. He explained that he does volunteer work at the hospital in the radiation ward, and that he tells the hospital doctors and nursing staff, every day, what a great job they are doing, and that he wakes up every morning being grateful to the medical profession for giving him another glorious day. Then he encouraged all of us to express our appreciation to our doctors and to make sure that they know they are appreciated. Then, right before my eyes, just about every one of those men whose early treatments had been ineffective (or the cancer wouldn't have returned) spoke up and reinforced the positive testimony of the facilitator. Although I had been an active participant earlier, I just sat there in mute disbelief and waited for the meeting to end.

Since then I have relived that session, honestly trying to determine the motivation for its approach. Granted that people who are experiencing cancer treatments and those who have reached the recovery phase need to function in a way that will enhance their chances of permanent success. I think there probably is a correlation between thinking you are getting well—and getting well. Conversely, I think there may be a correlation between being pessimistic and taking longer to heal or even failing to heal. However, I don't think you can fake optimism to any advantage. For me to become optimistic, I think I would need to have acquired some favorable results from my doctor's advice or treatment. Only then, I think, would I have a genuine basis for optimism.

The fact that I was appalled at what I witnessed in that support group didn't mean that I didn't recognize the value that a positive attitude could contribute to speeding up recovery and improving health. I knew it could, and I certainly hoped and expected to eventually reach that point. But, in the early stages of encountering cancer, I believe there are a number of well known psychological steps to work through before reaching "positive," and we don't all reach it at the same time. I certainly wasn't positive about anything at that point in my life.

16

RADIATION GRADUATION

(August 8, 1997)

On August 5th I completed my 35th treatment, which I originally thought would be my last. In the prior few days I had endured some rectum pain and minor bleeding. I was hopeful that this area of my body could hold up for just three more treatments without getting out of hand. I was scheduled for a conference with the doctor the next day. My one-hour session with the doctor was scheduled near the end of my treatments, scheduled specifically to allow me to get answers to any questions that I might have. I particularly wanted to know how much radiation would have been applied and how that amount was determined. He started out by explaining that my prostate was small, and with my relatively low PSA level (10) and Gleason score (5) he saw no need to radiate the lymph nodes. By making that decision, more of the dosage could be applied to the prostate, where the cancer was concentrated, and not wasted on an area thought to be cancer free. As a precaution, however, he did apply the first 25 radiation treatments to an area which included the seminal vesicles, which is soft tissue adjacent to the prostate. An average of 180 Rads (a measurement of energy) was applied at each of the first 25 treatments, totaling 4500 Rads. The final 13 treatments would be of 190 Rads each and would be targeted to the smaller area of just the prostate itself. These 13 treatments would consist of 2470 Rads, for a grand total of 6970 Rads. I had learned during my research that this level of radiation was slightly above average, so I was pleased. He further explained that by having applied hormonal therapy prior to and during radiation, my prostate and any cancer tumors will have shrunk, thus lessening the workload for the radiation. He had told me initially that he intended to apply radiation on the high side, and I believed that was what the three extra treatments would be, making a total of 38. Knowing that I would only get one shot at radiation, I wanted that extra punch. Dr. Bruce gave me the full hour and promised to supply me with copies of my medical tests and prescriptions, as well as negatives of the CT Scan. He was most generous with his time and his patience.

Friday, August 8, 1997 finally arrived. This was the day of my 38th and last treatment. I arrived a little early, to have more time to bid farewell to my waiting-room friends. Doris followed me in—she too was always early. I knew Randall would be early because this was also his last day. And my longer-term friend, Harold, whose wife, Ruby died during his treatments, was sitting there waiting for our usual morning talk. Just as he moved over so I could talk into his good ear, the therapist called his name. We hastily shook hands and bid each other farewell. Harold had two more radiation treatments and then was scheduled for Chemotherapy. The cancer of each of these three patients was in a much more critical stage than mine was. Harold's neck was red, as if from lying on the beach too long, and his throat was so raw he had difficulty eating. Randall had lung cancer and suffered a great deal from internal pain from his treatments—he had previously undergone Chemotherapy. Doris had throat cancer and had only recently begun her treatments—she had already lost her husband to cancer. It's amazing how heartfelt our concern for each other developed in such a short time.

My favorite therapist, Ron, called me for my last treatment. As he was lining up the marks on my body to the laser beams, I was already anticipating a vigorous shower without regard for eradicating the alignment marks. Then, as the linear accelerator was buzzing away, beaming its very last stream of destruction through my pelvis and into my prostate, I visualized the single remaining cancer cell getting zapped and gasping its last breath—then disintegrating and crumbling into the ruins of all the other smoldering cancer cells. The buzzing stopped for the last time. I swung off the table, pulled up my pants and gave Ron a hearty handshake, thanking him for his efforts on my behalf. Then I turned and walked away from round one of my fight against cancer.

On my drive home, it dawned on me that during the many days and weeks I had literally turned my life over to the medical professionals, not once had they made any nutritional recommendations, other than what not to eat during radiation. I had learned that nutrition wasn't even taught in medical schools in the past, and that now some schools teach just one three-hour course. It's very difficult to understand how doctors can isolate their practice from the field of nutrition and expect to provide the best medical care to their patients.

17

RETURNING TO CIVILIAN LIFE

The next few days were spent making up for the nutritional depriva-tion I had been experiencing for the last two months. First I ate a raw pear. Then I made sure a salad was on the menu for dinner. Of course we quickly reverted to whole-grain wheat bread and raw fruits and vegetables. A few days later the lunch I had with a friend included a martini on the rocks with two olives (I didn't count this as nutri-tional). Getting back to normal felt good—especially staying up later and getting to sleep longer.

During treatment I was instructed to avoid eating foods with high fiber content, which deprived me of the foods I enjoy the most. But in order to avoid weight loss, which normally occurs, I was encouraged to eat more of the kind of foods they prescribed. As a result, I didn't lose over two pounds and I maintained my strength quite well.

The hot flashes from hormone injections and pills were still occur-ring and interfering with my sleep, but hopefully this would wear off. The only other side effects I was experiencing were more frequent bowel movements and premature urgencies to urinate. I expected both of these problems to gradually fade away.

A month later I was still experiencing hot flashes, even though my last injection of Lupron had occurred 56 days prior (it was only a 30 day dosage). Also, I had been off of Casodex, the hormone pills, for 25 days. I had developed sympathy for women who experience hot flashes as they go through menopause, but, based on those I have questioned, mine were more frequent and were continuing over a much longer period than theirs. When my hot flash would start, I was instantly sweating and very uncomfortable. Then five or ten minutes later, when it stopped, even if everyone else was comfortable, I would be too cold for awhile. At night my sleep would be interrupted a number of times by hot flashes, and regardless of the temperature, my pajamas were wet from sweat. I hadn't bothered calling my radiologist because I had a routine appointment with him soon. I was certainly hoping that when I did meet with him, he would have a remedy for my problem.

During this "post-radiation" period, I had begun, in earnest, the study of nutritional supplements and vitamins. Not surprisingly, many of the books I reviewed seemed to have been written to sell books or to sell nutrition, as opposed to providing unbiased, objective recommendations. However, I was sure there was value in much of the material, and I tried to separate the "wheat from the chaff" and make the best choices I could in deciding which programs to follow.

On September 18, just six weeks after my last radiation treatment, I had my first follow-up meeting with my radiologist. We had a short discussion about how I was feeling and he told me that, thankfully, my hot flashes should soon disappear. He gave me a digital rectal exam and reported that the prostate was nice and smooth and had shrunk, just as it was supposed to. This was indeed good news. He also gave me a complete set of test results and medical records, which I had requested (I like to have my own copies so I can compare them with previous results). Dr. Bruce informed me that he would see me in one year, and that my urologist would be monitoring me quarterly for awhile. I would also be getting a PSA test within a month or so, which I presumed was for the purpose of comparison with later tests. I knew that after both surgery and radiation, regular PSA tests are given and used to monitor the success or failure of treatment. For prostate cancer patients, getting PSA tests on a regular basis, and sweating them out each time, would become a way of life.

I left blood for a PSA test at the end of October, and three days later I received a call from Dr. Bruce. He gave me the news that my test results were 0.22, which he said was lower than normal, and that, based on his experience, patients who test this low this early usually prove to be cancer free. I appreciated that doctor's personal call and his obvious interest and concern for me. But this news was tempered by information I had seen in a number of medical journals that largely discounted PSA tests taken sooner than a year after either surgery or radiation. By one year after radiation, if cancer has been cured, levels should stay below 1 or even below 0.5. If, however, readings start rising, certainly if they increase to 1 or 2, cancer has likely not been eradicated. But still I was encouraged, because I had gained considerable confidence in my doctor and didn't think he would deceive me. At the same time, I would really take the next test seriously.

By mid-January, 1998, five months since my last radiation treatment, my hot flashes had long since vanished, but my rectum damage still persisted. I remembered the words of a radiologist who spoke to a support group I had attended. He said, "regardless of what anyone else tells you, once you have had radiation therapy, your bowels will never be the same again." He was right. To escape some rectal damage from radiation treatment is apparently impossible because a small part of the rectum is adjacent to the prostate (separated by a layer of tissue that is about one eighth of an inch thick), so that area of the rectum will receive almost as much radiation as the prostate itself. In my case, the rectal irritation, or sensitivity, seemed to trigger bowel movements two or three times a day, instead of the normal once. Beyond this, I seemed to have more than normal gas built-up, which not only was uncomfortable, but also could prove embarrassing. On the other hand, eating healthier food, which included high fiber content foods, may have been contributing to that increased gas buildup.

I started a separate file for my prostate related medical bills, starting with my first trip to the urologist in February 1997. At the end of 1997, I reviewed and categorized all the bills from the various providers. The total cost so far (there would likely be more) was $20,317. My personal share was about $800, with Medicare and my secondary insurance paying the rest. The breakdown of the major expenses were Radiation therapy $13,414, Hormone injections $2582, Thallium stress test $1678. X-ray, CT Scan & Bone scan combined was $1809. These costs are the amounts billed by the providers before being adjusted downward by Medicare. Most of the suppliers accept assignment, which means they are paid a lower price than they bill. The only bill that I considered outrageous was $2582 for the four Lupron injections. When I discovered that just one 30-day injection costs $645, I couldn't believe it! The last time I had gone for my monthly injection, I asked the nurses who administered the serum what they thought it cost, and the highest guess was $35. They were genuinely astonished when I told them the actual cost.

18

CHANGING MY LIFESTYLE

❦

(1998)

In 1975 I was diagnosed with a clogged artery and had undergone bypass surgery. I was 50 years old. That was indeed a major event in my life, because up to then I thought I was indestructible. In my first 50 years I had survived a number of life-threatening experiences, including combat in World War II, and had come through relatively unscathed. Experiencing open-heart surgery brought me to an abrupt realization that I indeed was destructible. While recuperating, I began reassessing many aspects of my life, including how to take better care of my health. For the first time I started seeking out and listening seriously to advice about which foods to eat and which to avoid. The hospital provided a seminar on nutrition that was tailored to the heart patient. When I left the hospital, we started to gradually change our diet, and one of our first steps was to remove the sugar bowl and the salt shaker from the table. From then on, we ate whole wheat bread, and never had white bread in the house again until it was mandated during the course of my radiation treatments. Throughout the years, Peg and I have continued to seek nutritional advice and to modify our diet accordingly.

I had an Aunt who learned, when she was about 50, that she had a serious heart problem, and whatever her doctor was prescribing wasn't working. This, of course, was many years before by-pass surgery was practiced. She learned from a doctor, who may have been well ahead of his time, that she could be helped by taking massive doses of vitamin E. She used this supplement the rest of her life and enjoyed relatively good health well into her 70s. I learned about her experience while recovering from my heart surgery. I checked with my doctor and started taking vitamin E (but not massive doses). It wasn't until the mid-90s when I started noticing a tremendous increase in publicity about the many benefits of Vitamin E. I also had read how beneficial bran is in moving food through the digestive system more rapidly, so I added this to my diet. I started mixing bran and lecithin in a glass of orange juice and drinking it every day. Not only do I believe my heart benefited, but it also remedied a constipation problem that had plagued me off and on for years. I recognize that all patients are different, so I consult with my doctor before making a change in supplements.

When I had a minor heart attack in 1983, I took additional steps to take better care of myself. While still in the hospital I signed up for a hospital sponsored rehabilitation program that monitored me while I exercised on a treadmill or a stationary bicycle. When I completed that program I continued walking every day, and through 1998, I had logged over 11,000 miles. I certainly have my share of health problems, but according to my cardiologist, my cardiovascular system has improved substantially since 1983. I attribute much of this improvement to walking, which I will continue as long as possible.

Several months ago I started the process of learning everything I could about nutrition, and the foods and supplements that would benefit me the most in my defense against the return of cancer. It became apparent very early that nutrition is a confusing field of study. There are books galore on the subject but few are written by medical doctors. Believe it or not, their medical training curriculum, until recent years, hasn't included nutrition. Unfortunately, the medical schools traditionally have turned up their collective noses at the possibility that unconventional methods of treatment might have some merit. While the government has funded billions of dollars per year to the medical profession for conventional research, only a pittance has been made available for researching promising unconventional treatments such as nutritional supplements, herbal remedies, acupuncture and massage—just to name a few.

In 1990 members of the medical profession got the shock of their lives when the New England Journal of Medicine reported that 425 million visits were made to alternative care givers versus 388 million to primary care physicians. In 1992 the federal government responded to public pressure and directed the National Institute of Health to create the Office of Alternative Medicine, and provided the funding which, two years later, increased to 20 million dollars a year. Hopefully, funding will continue to increase to meet the demands of the rapidly increasing number of participants. This agency's purpose is to sponsor research, evaluate unconventional methods of curing and preventing diseases and to disseminate information to the public. Included in this research is the study and testing of the healing qualities of foods. Finally the process is in place, after all this wasted time, to eliminate a distinction between the terms "conventional" and "alternative" treatments, and start applying the most effective remedies available. It will be several years before we will start receiving direct benefits from this research. But when we do, I think the major benefit will be in learning which supplements and foods can be used not only to cure, but also to prevent illnesses.

In the meantime, without the results of unbiased nutritional research, l needed to do the best I could to establish an improved nutritional program. My overriding concern was to find the most effective way to fortify the immune system so it could better do its job in combating cancer. As a matter of fact, there is medical evidence that microscopic cancer cells routinely invade our bodies throughout our lives, and are quickly identified and routed (in most cases) by our immune systems. Therefore, eating the kinds of foods and taking the nutritional supplements that might help strengthen and fortify the immune system would surely be essential, especially to those of us who have already experienced cancer, because our immune system obviously wasn't up to the task of warding it off in the first place.

During 38 radiation treatments, my immune system undoubtedly suffered considerable damage and needed to be refortified. Even before I had progressed very far in the investigation of nutritional supplements, I had started altering my diet and taking additional vitamins and mineral supplements. As my research continued, and as I sought the advice of professionals who I believed were credible, I continued to make adjustments. I believed that following an optimum nutritional program just might add some years to my life.

A number of scientific studies have revealed that far fewer Japanese men die from PC than do men in the United States. What incomplete research reveals so far is that the Japanese diet consists of very little meat and is mainly vegetables. Even in cases where PC exists in men in Japan, it seems to progress more slowly, and is seldom responsible for deaths. Japanese men who have moved to the United States eventually die from PC at about the same rate as native Americans—seemingly because they adopt our diets.

At Sloan-Kettering Research Center, in an experiment with mice, they discovered that "it was difficult to grow prostate tumors in mice that ate low-fat diets." Their research also showed that growth of established tumors slows when the fat intake of animals is restricted. This correlates with the fact that eating too much fat directly increases testosterone levels in men, which increases the source of food for cancer cells, stimulating the growth of PC tumors.

Soy protein also seems to have an adverse effect on prostate cancer cells. Dr. Fair at Sloan Kettering reported, "If we add soy protein in the medium in which the cells are growing, we markedly inhibit growth. In fact, most of the cells die. In addition, when soy is fed to mice that have PC, tumor growth slows down or stops growing."

Japanese men eat a lot of soy, far more than do American men, and this is thought to be a major factor in their low death rate from PC. The fact that they eat very little meat may also be a factor.

Frequently my relatives and friends had been asking how I was holding up to the pain and anguish of my cancer problem. It was difficult responding to their concern without explaining in more detail than they would want to hear. Although I had explained previously that I had suffered no pain, even during radiation treatment, it didn't seem to have registered. I really didn't want to burden anyone with my real concerns: that choosing radiation treatment may have been the wrong course of action, that the equipment used may not have been the best choice, that there may have been errors made in the process of administering the 38 treatments, or that treatment may not have been started in time. Those are concerns that I will always live with, as do all cancer patients. So, although I was thankful for the concern of others, I sensed their discomfort in talking about it—and they likely sensed mine.

One morning I encountered a friend I hadn't seen for awhile. After acknowledging that I was getting along all right with my cancer problem, he shared the experience his father had with prostate cancer back in the 1970s. He had worked all his life as an accountant, and had looked forward to early retirement because he so enjoyed a number of hobbies, including gardening. His prostate was removed surgically, which left him both impotent and incontinent (requiring him to wear a urination bag). Well beyond the time required for physical healing from the operation, he just sat around the house feeling sorry for himself. It wasn't until his wife practically threatened to leave him that he came to his senses. He went to work in the garden growing things, which he loved to do. In the process he gained his zest for life. As he explained to his family, he finally realized that living with the ravages of an operation was certainly better than the alternative—and he lived into his eighties before dying from a stroke.

In the spring of 1998, eight months after my radiation treatments, I had settled down to the following "lifestyle" program in my effort to enhance my health and well being. The regimen was based on what I had learned in the past, coupled with information gleaned from recent research. My aim was to keep myself reasonably slender, to maintain the optimum HDL/LDL cholesterol ratio, and to build up my immune system. I decided to emphasize exercise, diet, nutritional supplements, stimulating physical and mental activity:

Exercise consisted of walking not less than two miles daily at the rate of 15 minutes per mile. I would follow this up with a series of upper body exercises using a Rider exercise machine and doing a series of floor exercises.

Diet: We had eliminated at least 70 per cent of red meat and fatty foods such as French fries, eggs, fried food of any kind and all organ meats. We would use only skim milk, whole grain wheat breads, baked fish and skinned broiled chicken. We ate a wide range of soups, all homemade so we could control the sodium and fat. We ate generous quantities of vegetables and fruit daily. We had added soybean products to our diet and alternated between tofu, soymilk and lecithin, to maintain our protein input requirement. We kept adjusting what we ate as we gained more knowledge.

Nutritional Supplements: We would change the strength and the frequencies, and sometimes the supplements as we acquired more knowledge. However, we constantly recognized that we couldn't verify the reliability of any of our selections, and would never make recommendations to others. At one point, these are the supplements we were taking, and for the reasons as stated by various sources:

Zinc: important in strengthening the immune system, stabilizes membranes, enhances wound healing and aids in the re-growth of tissue after radiation has damaged it. Food sources include nuts, whole grains, split pea, lima beans, sardines, haddock, potatoes, lecithin and garlic.

Selenium: may inhibit the formation and growth of tumors by improving the body's defenses against free radicals. May be toxic to tumors. Works synergistically with vitamin E to protect the lipids in cell membranes. Food sources include Brazil nuts, swordfish, salmon, tuna, haddock, sunflower seed, barley and rice.

Vitamin E: An antioxidant. Works with Vitamin C in protecting the lipids in the cells. Protects healthy cells from some of the toxicity of radiation and stimulates the immune system. Food sources include eggs, organ meat, wheat germ, soybeans, dark green vegetables, brown rice and butter.

Multivitamin/Multi-mineral Supplement: I chose one that was tailored to over 50+. This was one way to insure that I was getting at least the minimal requirements of essential minerals and vitamins.

Garlic: A natural antibiotic that helps stave off bacterial and viral infection and block tumor growth. It also is credited with reducing cholesterol.

19

HAUNTED BY RADIATION DAMAGE

✦

(May 1998)

I had an appointment for a routine consultation with Dr. Stevens, my regular doctor. The good news was that my cholesterol tested 159, with a favorable LDL/HDL ratio of 3.0. Zocor, a prescription drug to lower cholesterol, warranted most of the credit, but I was confident my eating and exercise habits helped. We talked about the status of my prostate and I described the only remaining problem I was experiencing. In the past my normal routine was to have one bowel movement a day. Since radiation, I was experiencing two or three a day, plus occasional urgencies which turned out to be false. In addition, I had an unusual amount of gas build up, which bothered me. He said that this was a typical problem, because radiation almost always resulted in some damage to the rectum. It also had probably damaged the ligaments and nerves of the sphincter, which controls bowel movement. I confessed that having more than one bowel movement a day wasn't all that bad, but I was more concerned about body odor which two showers a day didn't always remedy. His reply to this was a little disheartening. He said the odor is likely coming from minor leaking which can only be remedied by wearing special pads. His final hopeful comment was that this condition would usually return to normal within a year or two.

On May 19, 1998, I left blood for my second post-surgery PSA test and two weeks later had my routine follow-up visit with my urologist. I already had a copy of my test results and knew that it tested 0.17, a decline from my 0.22 six months earlier. The doctor was equally satisfied with the test results. He told me that a few years ago post-radiation PSA results below 1.0 to 1.5 were considered satisfactory. Now standards have been lowered to the area of 0.5. My extremely low score, plus the fact that I was feeling fine and not suffering any pain or energy loss was apparently justification for optimism. He gave me my routine digital prostate and rectum exam and asked me to schedule another visit in six months.

A year and a half ago, when I had attended my World War II, 65th Division Association reunion for the first time, I was asked to accept one of the offices on the executive committee, and I had declined. At that time I had just received my high PSA test results and was too pessimistic to think that I should take on that kind of responsibility. Then, a year later, after going through radiation therapy and becoming more optimistic about my future, I had accepted the appointment as editor of our division magazine. In this job I was in frequent contact with our president, who just a few weeks later advised me that he had a positive biopsy for prostate cancer. He was 72, the same age I was when I received the same diagnosis. About two weeks later, our second Vice President learned that his PSA test was high and he was scheduled for a biopsy. I guess there was really nothing surprising about the fact that every veteran of WW II is over 70, thus a prime candidate for prostate cancer.

On July 8, my 74th birthday, I noticed some blood in my stool. According to my research, the number of men who experience bleeding after radiation treatment is only about 5 in 100. This bleeding is painless and usually occurs when I am having a bowel movement. But if it persists, it can lead to complications, one of which can result in the need for a colostomy (surgical formation of an artificial anus). Also, bleeding can be a symptom of colon cancer. In either case, after what I had been through so far, I had no intention of delaying getting this problem checked out.

I called Dr. Steven's secretary, explained my problem and asked her to get the doctor to refer me to the appropriate specialist. After she provided me the name of a specialist, it took some pretty intensive persuasion to secure an appointment within a reasonable period of time. I wasn't about to accept the frustrating routine of a long wait for an appointment to deal with what might be a very high priority problem—and one where weeks, or even days, could make a difference. I was fortunate to get an appointment one-week out due to a cancellation.

On July 13 I had a 30-minute conference with Dr. Crompton, the Gastroenterology Specialist who Dr. Stevens had recommended. We discussed my concerns and got right to my problem of blood on the stool. He agreed that this was definitely the symptom of a problem, even though I wasn't experiencing any intestinal pain or discomfort. And in answer to my question, eating lots of raw fruit and vegetables and taking bran would definitely not be causing the blood. After reviewing my medical history, he stated that the likelihood of my having cancer in the colon was greater because I already had cancer in my system, plus the genetic consequence of my mother, my sister and a brother all dying of cancer.

He said that a colonoscopy should be performed, and that it was an extensive process, which had some risks, and that it would require me to be anesthetized. He explained that a colonoscopy involved inserting a lubricated flexible colonoscope into the rectum and then advancing it slowly through the entire colon. This would allow him to visually and thoroughly examine the bowel lining of the entire large intestine (colon). If polyps were present, he would remove them during the colonoscopy by electrocautery. If he encountered any suspicious areas, he would take off tissue samples during the course of the procedure, which would be biopsyed within a few days right in the hospital. After I consented to the procedure, he carefully reviewed the preparation instructions I would need to follow the two days prior to the colonos-copy. We made an appointment to have this procedure performed the following week. We were leaving the next day on a trip. I didn't expect that this trip would make me forget what was at stake when I got back, but maybe it would take my mind off of it for awhile.

During this entire prostate cancer journey, I've had qualms at every turn. I had developed a small boil on the back of my neck, and every time I felt it, I wondered if it was malignant. A year or so ago I had a "pre-cancerous" tissue removed from my face, and sometimes when I shaved, that spot seemed to feel a little tender, and I wondered if it was coming back. I'd had two PSA tests since my radiation treatments, and I was uneasy both times while I waited the normal interminable amount of time for the results. I'm sure this process will continue for the rest of my life. Now I was facing the prospects of a problem that had the potential of being even more threatening than prostate can-cer—colon cancer.

Dr. Crompton, I would guess, was in his early 40's and appeared to be a competent professional. He certainly had a pleasing personality, and was easy to like. But during this first and only session, I didn't detect more than a hint of empathy on his part to my gut-wrenching anxiety about the possible consequences I was facing. Perhaps I mis-read him. Maybe I was just concealing my "apprehension signals," so they were invisible to him. But on the other hand, what should I have expected. With all the specialists that exist today, patients are con-stantly meeting them for the first time. It isn't like it used to be when the family doctor did it all, and, over time, became almost like a mem-ber of the family. They would always respond to the mood of their patients the minute they walked through the door. Times have changed, dramatically.

During the past week I had spent too much time remembering back when I was sweating out the results of my prostate biopsy, hoping against hope that it was negative. But it wasn't. Then, with this proce-dure, I felt like I was repeating my worst nightmare. I had no concern about the procedure itself, about the two days of fasting or any pain that might be involved. I just wanted whatever he cut out of my colon to result in a negative biopsy report—because if it didn't, I knew I would be in dire trouble.

At that time I had lived over a year as a cancer victim and had developed kind of a fatalistic attitude when any setback occurred. It was as if I no longer had any control over what would happen to me. This much lack of control seemed different than anything I had ever experienced. Before, if I had played a bad game of golf, I was despondent, but I could at least hope to do better the next time. If I had gained too much weight, I could eat less and exercise more to solve that problem. When I had injuries, like a dislocated shoulder, or a bad burn, the proper treatment would quickly get me on the way to a complete recovery. Even when fighting a war, I could keep my head down as the bullets came and dig my foxhole deeper to survive the artillery barrages. But at 74, with prostate cancer, options vanished. I seemed to be at the mercy of whatever setbacks came along.

We arrived at the Endoscopy Department of the hospital and within a few minutes I was registered in and escorted to a dressing room. I quickly changed into a hospital gown and then occupied a bed in the preparation room. A very pleasant nurse reviewed my status, asked a few questions and made notes of my answers and then answered any questions I had. I was hooked up to an IV in preparation for my colonoscopy procedure. I was wheeled into a nearby room where the procedure would take place. Nurses moved me near the monitor and positioned me properly on the gurney. Dr. Crompton walked in, verified that I had followed all of the pre-operation procedures of fasting and taking the required substances to clean out my colon, and proceeded to go to work. He turned a valve and told me that he was now administrating the Demerol and that I would feel some numbness. Almost before he finished talking, I felt a strong surge of numbness—and that's the last I remember. I woke up in the preparation area about an hour later.

After the procedure, while I was recovering, the doctor had visited with Peg and given her a file of material for me to review. He had told her that he hadn't seen anything suspicious so he hadn't taken any tissue samples to biopsy. He informed her that the blood appeared to be coming from some inflammation of the rectum, which was apparently damaged from radiation. I was to insert a Mesalamine suppository in my rectum daily at bedtime, and call him in 10 days to report on the results. I was so elated to learn that I didn't have cancer of the colon that, at that moment, my concern about having an inflamed rectum that wouldn't heal had vanished.

During this period that I was taking suppositories to combat the rectal bleeding, I referred to some of the research material I had accumulated about radiation rectum damage. It stated that when rectal damage does occur, it is usually six to 24 months after completing radiation treatments before it starts bleeding. "The delay is due to the time required for the radiation-related weakening of the rectum tissue to develop." At that time, it had been exactly one year since I had finished my treatments. But it also verified that damage to the rectum was the most serious, but uncommon, complication of radiation. My research further revealed that the rectum of some patients would not tolerate the radiation and those patients might develop inflammation which could lead to rectal bleeding. The bleeding would be painless and would usually occur when having a bowel movement, and was caused by the pressure from the stool passing through the rectum. The one hopeful comment in one reference was that such bleeding would usually stop spontaneously within one to three years, and that medication may help this condition to heal faster. There was also a remote chance (less than 1%) that bleeding could become excessive and would not stop. In some cases, a colostomy might be required. The prospects of having to resort to this remedy was so repugnant to me that I would try very hard to dismiss it from my mind.

During the course of these 10 days I made sure to use a suppository each night and to examine my stool for blood the next morning. I wanted to be sure to convey accurate information to Dr. Crompton. When I did report to him that I was seeing blood about a third of the time, he merely phoned in a prescription for another 12 suppositories, explaining that it sometimes takes longer to get the desired results.

During the next 10 days, results were about the same. This time he changed me to a different suppository and had me take it two times daily, night and morning. When it was time to turn in a report of these results I had to tell him that there was no apparent change, that blood was apparent about 30 percent of the time. Again he sent more prescriptions, and asked me to experiment between one and two per day to see what difference it would make. Apparently this would be an ongoing effort. All of my contacts since the colonoscopy were by telephone, in most cases with his assistant. I was uncomfortable, not getting the full story of what to expect long-term. However I would be having a discussion with my radiologist the following month and could get his opinion. In my minds eye, I pictured a 2 to 3 cm area of my rectum as raw flesh, with destroyed vessel endings and dying tissue beginning to decay, with chances of reinvigoration diminishing daily. It was not a pretty sight.

20

STILL A LONG WAY TO GO

An important and time-consuming activity for me since February 1997 was editing my world war division semi-annual magazine. This job was demanding and time consuming, especially at first, but it helped keep my mind off of my health problems. As the editor, I was in close contact with our president, Jack Rheiner, and we had become good friends. So I was devastated when he called and told me that he just discovered that he also had prostate cancer.

Soon after his positive biopsy, he began having considerable pain in his rib area, and this led to a bone scan, which was negative. After that, since there was some chance that the cancer had spread beyond the prostate area, he went through the very painful process of having his lymph nodes surgically removed and biopsied. This procedure is very seldom done, but Jack was willing to endure the pain in order to help make a better treatment decision. After sweating these results out for a week, he was much relieved to get a negative report (presumably no cancer in his lymph nodes, which should mean that cancer hadn't spread beyond the prostate). In the meantime, he had been on hormone treatment, just as I was, intending to wait until after our division convention in September to start his radiation treatments. About a week before the convention, Jack informed me that the pain in his rib area had flared up again and his physician had him scheduled for another scan. Then he called later and told me that this time, he got a positive result, indicating that cancer had spread to the bone. In spite of that dire diagnosis, he was bound and determined to attend the convention. His tenacity was unbelievable, and heart rendering. His diagnosis was obviously the worst possible news a prostate cancer patient could receive. There was nothing I could say to console him. In the past six months we had talked dozens of times on the phone. This time I was speechless. I must have stuttered and stammered, trying to think of something appropriate to say. As we ended that conversation, I was in so much pain emotionally that I hurt physically.

We arrived at the convention on schedule, and were relieved to see that Jack was there. Unfortunately, his news wasn't any better, and he confided to me that he knew he was in serious trouble. He had changed his schedule around so he could attend the convention, and he would be starting a series of tests, and maybe treatments, when he returned home. In the meantime, he was the president of our association, and he was in charge of the three-day convention. He didn't want to shirk his duties by dumping the workload on his vice-president. I knew he had been on hormonal treatment for several months, and that the hot flashes would have interrupted his sleep at night, just as they had mine. In addition, he was enduring a lot of pain with his cancer-infested rib area. The strain was apparent in his face.

However, as he conducted our executive committee meeting, and then the three-hour membership meeting the next day, he was magnificent. He must have utilized every ounce of fuel he had in his tank. Once our convention was over, I knew he would get right back on track with his doctors, going through further tests and probably starting on chemotherapy. I was just praying that when I would talk to him the next time, something miraculous would have occurred, and he would explain it to me with his customary enthusiasm.

I met with my Radiologist, Dr. Bruce. It had been just about a year since I last saw him. He made his usual digital examination of my prostate and said that there was no problem there. We discussed my current problem with bleeding of the rectum caused from radiation damage. I told him that suppositories weren't doing any good, and wondered if I should be concerned about the amount of blood I was losing. I also asked if I should be taking an iron supplement and he agreed that it wouldn't hurt. He gave me a prescription for a blood test to determine if there was any sign of anemia. If bleeding hasn't stopped within a month, he would likely recommend that Dr. Crompton cauterize the blood vessels that were damaged and were causing the bleeding. This was a relatively simple process, he said, and almost always cures the problem. However, I wanted to avoid any more "procedures," because I had learned that there was always a down side to a "procedure." I felt somewhat better after this visit, just knowing that there was a rather simple remedy for my blood loss, even if suppositories don't work. Ironically, during the week after that visit, I experienced practically no bleeding.

Just a week after returning from our division convention I just couldn't get my friend Jack Rheiner off my mind. Before he left for the convention, he had been told that his cancer had advanced to his bones. At the convention we spoke about it for just a moment, and he knew he had a serious problem. When a letter arrived from Jack, I knew the news would be bad. I read, "yesterday I received horrible news when I visited the University of Pennsylvania hospital. The oncologist said that even though I had a clear indication four months ago, my bones are now on fire with cancer cells."

I felt like I had been hit by a truck. Momentarily I couldn't finish the letter, and I felt goose bumps spread over my entire body. I knew he was in trouble, but the force and vividness of words like "on fire with cancer cells" was the strongest and most painful words I've ever read. I felt deep compassion, yet I knew there was absolutely nothing I could do or say to alter the path that Jack was destined to follow as he inevitably would lose his bout with prostate cancer. He was understandably in deep depression but was set on continuing to fulfill his responsibilities as president of our world war II Association. As I talked to him on the phone, he indicated that he was already using a cane to counteract his instability, caused from the deterioration of his cancer-ridden bone structure. He stated that he was purposely working hard on 65th Division business in order to keep his mind off of himself. His goals were to make it to our convention in Orlando in February 1999, and to complete his term as president at our 1999 fall convention in Biloxi, Mississippi. In the meantime, he was scheduled to go through another battery of tests, in a few days, which would determine if there was any treatment they would recommend.

The sad and troubling aspect of the status of Jack's prostate cancer was that less than eight months before, he had told me that his PSA tested 3.6. Based on my research and discussions with doctors, this was a pretty normal reading for a 72-year-old man. A reading of 3.6 would, at most, have indicated the very beginning of detectable cancer. Yet, in this case, he not only had cancer in his prostate, but it had likely already moved far beyond. In fact, it seems reasonable to assume that a year or two before, when the PSA test might have been 2.6, he may well have had cancer confined to the prostate, but that test score wouldn't have been high enough to suggest the need for a biopsy.

21

THE MEDICAL TESTING PROCESS

Here we were, in the fall of 1998, and about the only significant innovation to result from research of prostate cancer in the past 20 years was the PSA test. And still my friend Jack's life was in dire jeopardy because even that remarkable lifesaving discovery didn't work right for him.

The more I look for evidence of significant progress in dealing with prostate cancer, the less I find. Through the years I have read newspaper reports of new and miraculous medical discoveries, and like most people I know, I assumed that great progress in the medical field was being made. Now I have become more skeptical, not just of the research laboratories where these articles originate, but of the news reporters whose articles tend to convey overly optimistic expectations to the public. Every time these articles appear, doctors are flooded with calls from patients, expecting this new treatment to be applicable to their problem. Of course, it never is. I recently read an article that explained why these announcements, more times than not, are overblown and premature.

After a medical research institution has discovered a new drug that they think has potential, it has to go through three testing phases before it gets FDA approval. In phase I, it is extensively tested on animals first, then on humans, primarily to determine the harmful effects it has. Only about half of all cancer agents make it past phase I. Of those that do, 70% flunk phase II.

The extensive tests in phase II are performed on both animals and humans to measure how effectively the cancer agent does what it is designed to do. At the conclusion of this phase, the number of surviving agents has dwindled. During phase III the treatment is applied on at least 300 human patients. At this point researchers look to see if the agent actually works better than existing therapies. Since each testing phase takes considerable time, by the completion of phase III, side effects are known and claims of good results are quite reliable. The final step is approval of the FDA. Obviously if the medical research institutions would wait until new discoveries have at least passed phase II testing before it is reported in newspapers, the public would be better served. As long as the public is satisfied with medical progress, their motivation to push for improvement is diminished.

Most of us who have been informed that we have prostate cancer have probably paid much attention to this disease for the first time. In the process, we have each been shocked to learn that PC doesn't have as good a menu of solutions as we would have anticipated. We wouldn't have, in our wildest imagination, predicted how severe and harmful some of the consequences might be, regardless of the treatment choice. PC has often been referred to as the "silent disease," because, in the initial stages, it doesn't hurt. Consequently men are not reminded to do anything about it because they don't know they have it. And when they do learn that they have the problem, they tend to keep it to themselves, because it's a "masculinity thing." It is because men have historically kept it to themselves that may account for prostate cancer receiving less attention from the medical profession than is due. The worn out cliché, "the squeaky wheel gets the grease" is woefully appropriate when it comes to influencing those people in Washington who dispense funding for cancer research. Only in the last year or two have a large number of famous men such as Arnold Palmer, General Schwartzkopf, Bob Dole, Sam Donaldson and Mayor Rudolph Guilliani come forward to publicize their prostate cancer and to promote the need for more prostate cancer research. They also are emphasizing the importance of men over 50 getting annual PSA tests, and the response is great. Now, for the first time, prostate cancer is openly discussed on the airwaves and in the homes.

It is reported that 180,000 men in the year 2000 will discover that they have PC. Now is the time for all of us to get the message to Washington that we want more money appropriated to cancer research in order to speed up the discovery of a cure for PC. A few years ago women got organized and clamored for more funding for breast cancer research. Their voices were heard and their effort was so successful in getting government funding that today twice as much funding is directed to breast cancer than to prostate cancer. Yet, PC claims nearly the same number of lives each year as breast cancer and has the same survival rate if caught early. The public needs to take its head out of the sand and demand that government funding for all cancer be boosted substantially, every year, until we get it conquered!

In mid-October, 1998, my PSA test result was 0.2 ng/ml. That was my third test since I had completed radiation treatments 14 months earlier. Even though my previous tests had also been 0.2, this was the most comforting result because it was taken more than a year after treatment, which some research specialists say is the first post-treatment test that is meaningful. One research report states, "If cancer is destroyed by radiation, PSA should fall to very low levels within one year. If it is 1.0 or lower then, it likely is permanently eradicated." Recently, however, I have read where this standard has been lowered from 1.0 down to 0.5. In either case, being at 0.2 is where I was and where I hoped to stay.

On November 18, I learned that Jack Rheiner had fallen out of bed and broken his hip, and while hospitalized, had developed pneumonia. These two setbacks, along with his already fragile cancer-ridden condition, left him with no hope at all for survival. His wife conceded that he wasn't expected to live very long. And to think that only about eight weeks ago, he presided over our division convention in such a profes-

sional and energetic way that you would have thought he was indestructible.

On November 23, 1998, Jack Rheiner lost his courageous battle
with prostate cancer. He died just seven months after getting a PSA
test reading of 3.6 and having a prostate biopsy, which was positive.
His experience contradicted a number of things I had researched about
PSA test results defining prostate cancer staging. With a PSA reading
of 3.6, cancer would normally be confined to the prostate, where it
could be more likely treated successfully. In fact, that is precisely why
men are encouraged to get regular PSA tests, to detect cancer when it is
in its early stages, which a low score of 3.6 would indicate. But in this
case, at the time of the PSA test, the cancer cells had obviously already
spread beyond the prostate itself, in contradiction to the low test
results. Perhaps this was an uncommon exception to the normal test
results or maybe the testing itself was faulty. We'll never know.
Another aspect of this case was also difficult to understand. Before
prostate cancer reaches the bone, it usually has entered the lymph
nodes. Yet, four months after Jack got an all clear MRI bone scan and
lymph node biopsy, cancer was detected throughout his entire bone
structure. At that point, he was terminal. This case was especially
heartrending to me because I had assumed that his cancer had been
detected earlier than mine, and that he would be all right. Since we
were working so closely together as officers of our WWII 65th Division
Association, we were good friends. The fact that we had a common ail-
ment also brought us more closely together, because we were continu-
ously exchanging information about our respective treatments. Even
though I had known Jack Rheiner for less than a year, I will feel the
pain of his passing for the rest of my life. His unfortunate bout with
prostate cancer has already intensified my determination to do all I can
to publicize the urgent need for more Federal funds to be directed to
prostate cancer research.

By anyone's standard, it is inexcusable that we are still utilizing
archaic methods to deal with a disease that accounted for 40,000

deaths in 1998. In 1997, only about $2700 was spent on prostate cancer research for each death from the disease, while spending for breast cancer research totaled $12,800 per each death. Investment in Aids research totaled $47,000 per death. A recent journal reported that 180,000 men would learn that they have prostate cancer in the next 12 months. Unfortunately, funds for prostate cancer research is not even coming close to keeping up with the ever increasing numbers of men being diagnosed with the disease. Consequently, prostate cancer patients are continuing to be treated by surgery or radiation, the same archaic methods commonly used for the last 30 years. Massive increases in funding is needed now to accelerate the development of a number of promising innovations, any one of which may be the breakthrough that is needed.

22

PROGRESS ON THE HORIZON

There are a number of promising and exciting theories that cry out for accelerated development and research that have recently been publicized. The answer could well be among the following:

Anti-Angiogenesis Therapies: Stop prostate cancer by blocking the vessels that supply blood to the cancer tumors, allowing the cells to die.

Gene Therapies: Identifying the abnormal genes that make a cell cancerous, then develop a drug to either normalize it or kill it.

Immune Therapies: Our immune system is designed to protect the body against disease. Discover vaccines and stimulatory growth factors, which will enable the body's defense system to recognize and destroy cancer cells.

Nutrition Therapy: Determine the role of specific foods, vitamins and dietary supplements to aid in the fight against prostate cancer.

Therapies Targeting Metastasis: Prostate cancer becomes deadly only after it has spread outside the gland and into the rest of the body. This is an attempt to control the disease by preventing its spread to other organs, particularly bone.

These are just a few of the therapies that are being actively researched by Cap Cure, a privately financed effort started by Michael Milken. He is the financier who made millions in the stock market but in the process got into legal trouble and spent some time in prison. He is very wealthy and very bright. When he discovered that he had prostate cancer, he learned very quickly how inadequate our current alternatives were to deal with it. He decided to spearhead an effort to do something about it and spent over 50 million dollars to start CAP CURE, an association dedicated exclusively to finding a cure for cancer of the prostate. It has actively secured the services of some of the brightest scientists in the country and is gaining recognition and funding from all over the world. It takes considerable funding and many years of trial and error to develop and perfect, plus secure approval for a new therapy. None of these will likely help those of us who are presently undergoing therapy. But, by accelerating research now, any one of these therapies, or others, may be the one to win the war against prostate cancer for our children.

I recently read Tom Brokaw's book, "The Greatest Generation." This outstanding book emphasizes the significance of growing up during the great depression and participating in World War II, and how these experiences influenced the later accomplishments of that generation. It struck me, as I was reading, that the youngest WW II soldier alive in 1999 would be 73 and the oldest in his 90s. I have learned, through my work as editor of my division's news magazine, that a very high percentage of our members have experienced prostate problems. Our president, who was just 72, died from it eight months after he was biopsied. His successor had his cancerous prostate surgically removed 11 years ago. The second VP recently had an elevated PSA test result. When I talk to members, which I do on a continuing basis, I discover that prostate cancer is the most prevalent health problem among us. It's disheartening to realize all the pain and suffering and frustration that my generation is suffering and will suffer because of prostate cancer. Of all the great achievements we are given credit for, it's ironic that finding a cure for prostate cancer can't be counted among them. Hopefully, our children's generation will find not only the cure, but the prevention.

Recently I received a Christmas card from a relative of mine. He included a short note where he casually mentioned that he had recently had an elevated PSA test result. The impact this had on me was anything but mild. A week or so later I made a point to give him a call to see how he was doing and to reassure myself that he was taking that PSA test seriously. When I asked what his test score was, he replied that he didn't know, that the doctor just said it was elevated and that they would check it again in six months. I suggested that he might want to consult a urologist. This is when he hit me with, "why should I listen to your advice, you're not a doctor. I have confidence in my doctor. Whatever he tells me to do, I'll do. My doctor certainly didn't seem to be concerned about it and that's good enough for me." I was flabbergasted and irritated at that response, so I proceeded to change the subject. Later, I realized that he was merely into his early denial phase, just as I was when I got my elevated PSA test results. Hopefully, he will hear from someone he'll listen to, or come around on his own, and consult a urologist before it is too late.

I make a practice of talking to other men about my experience with prostate cancer. I particularly advise them about PSA testing and let them know how important it is for early detection. I also explain that prostate cancer, in its early stages, is a "silent" disease—it doesn't hurt—it doesn't cause any symptoms that you can feel—it's painless, so it can sneak up on you like it did on me. And in some cases I let them know that if it isn't detected and treated early, it will become terminal. It doesn't surprise me that just about everyone I talk to who hasn't already had a prostate problem doesn't know anything about it. In most cases, they have never had a PSA test and don't know what it is. Their lack of knowledge or concern is just about as deficient as mine was before I "got educated."

Traditionally, men don't like to talk about having prostate cancer. It is amazing how many people I have known for years and didn't know they had had a prostate cancer problem until I told them about mine. I guess their reluctance to discuss it comes from seeing prostate cancer as a threat to their masculinity. Unfortunately, this reluctance has probably been a contributing factor to the lack of more funding for prostate cancer research. If the wheel doesn't squeak, it doesn't get greased!

The biggest problem in dealing with cancer is the inability to detect it in its earliest stages. As near as I can determine, every instrument or test we use for this purpose can only detect cancer cells after they have developed to a certain mass. A urologist told me recently that cancer couldn't be detected by any devices yet invented until it contains at least one billion cells. At that point it is the size of a pea and is about the weight of a paperclip. By then, it has been in the body for several years. Even after it is detected, we are still unable, with any certainty, to determine how far the cancer cells have advanced in the body. Oh there are clues, but they are not definitive. When they are discovered, they have more than likely been minuscule cancer cells earlier, and prior to that, "pre-malignant cells" (cells in the process of becoming cancerous). Hopefully, research in the area of earlier detection will come soon. I read recently where scientists at one hospital have discovered that there are two types of prostate cancer: one carries more of a protein called p27—a cell inhibitor that suppresses tumor growth. They discovered that cancers with lower levels of p27 were more aggressive. This discovery should lead to adding this test at the time of biopsies in order to facilitate determining how aggressive the treatment needs to be. There was no indication of when this additional test will be available. Also, if anyone is getting close to being able to detect prostate cancer when it is at the pre-malignancy stage, or just after, I haven't heard about it.

In mid-March, 1999, it had been 19 months since I finished my radiation treatments. I had received three consistently favorable PSA tests (0.2 or below) and had gradually begun to feel optimistic about my future. In the past year I had communicated with a large number of veterans who were in my division in WWII. The ages of these men run from 73 to the high 80s. From these phone calls I have learned that a very high percentage are being treated for a prostate problem, or have been in the past. I guess it isn't surprising that if you live long enough, you'll become unhealthy.

Just after the new year, 1999, I learned that Gary Miesse, a very special friend of mine who lives in South Carolina, had been diagnosed with prostate cancer. This really floored me. He was just 57 and seemingly in great physical shape. He had always exercised regularly and had received annual physicals for as long as I had known him. He was first tested in 1991 and had a PSA of 1.8. His next test recorded 1.5 in 1993, 3.0 in 1997, 3.1 in January 1998 and 3.4 in August 1998. Fortunately for him, his doctor was skeptical enough to refer him to a urologist. The biopsy revealed cancer in one tissue sample in just one lobe, and the cancer was presumed to be confined to the prostate. Hormonal treatment was started immediately, and surgery was performed on February 5, 1999. The lymph nodes and seminal vesicles were removed along with the prostate and, as is a common practice, everything that was removed was retained and placed under the microscope. It was several weeks before Gary got the results of the post-surgery biopsy. The lymph nodes and seminal vesicles tested negative, but cancer was found in both lodes of the prostate (the biopsy prior to surgery revealed cancer in only one). In addition, the pathologist discovered a hole in one of the tumor capsules. This "red flag" discovery would seem to open up the possibility that cancer cells escaped into the body beyond the confines of the prostate. This would be devastating.

The first post-operation PSA test would be made eight weeks out. I doubted if there was any way on earth to ascertain if, in fact, a cancer cell had escaped. Even if they knew it had, additional treatment, such as radiation, couldn't be performed until the healing process from the operation had occurred. In the meantime, everyone involved would be sweating each successive PSA test result, which every prostate cancer patient would be doing for the rest of his life. Another nagging concern for Gary was the apparent fact that the younger you are when you have prostate cancer, the more aggressive are the cancer cells. Gary and his family are on a journey down a bumpy road laden with many unknown twists and turns.

On April 3, 1999 Gary called with the results of his first PSA test since his surgery about seven weeks prior. He was scheduled to see his Urologist in a few days and wanted his test results before this visit. He told me that he tested 0.1. This news hit me like a bowling ball in the stomach. Even while we continued to talk, I had a flashback to when I first scheduled an appointment with my Urologist after having my high PSA test in 1997. He was a little delayed coming into the office where I was waiting for our initial conference prior to scheduling my biopsy procedure. When my doctor did walk in he looked troubled. After introducing himself, he seemed compelled to share his problem with me, even though we weren't even acquainted yet. He had just finished talking to a patient he had operated on about a year before, and whose PSA tests had been negative ever since the operation—except for the one he had just received. It had tested 0.1, which was a clear indication that cancer had recurred. It was the very worst news that could be given to a cancer patient who had his prostate removed, because the only reason for removing the prostate is to remove all of the cancer cells. My sympathy went out to that patient and I immediately gained respect for my urologist for being so affected by this unsettling news.

I desperately hoped that Gary's test result wasn't a repeat of that patient of Dr. Callon's. I could only hope that it was a bad test, which does happen, or that the test was given too soon after the operation to be valid. As I continued to talk to Gary he indicated that the doctor wasn't concerned, and that he even indicated that it was an unusually low reading so soon after the surgery. He also reiterated that a reading of 0.1 actually means zero to 0.1 because that's as precise as they can measure. I didn't challenge this explanation with Gary and we concluded our visit on a high note. However, in my own mind I was concerned because this explanation didn't coincide with what I had learned from my research or with the experience my urologist shared with me. Gary and I call each other every few months, and I was already sweating out our next conversation.

23

RESEARCH CONCLUSIONS

In May 1999, a full-page, single column article from the Associated Press appeared on the front page of our newspaper titled "Relief To Cancer Patients." It was based on a recent article from the Journal of the American Medical Association (JAMA). Since newspaper articles are so often misleadingly positive, as this was, I made a point to get my hands on the original research, which came from Johns Hopkins Hospital and is titled "Natural History of Progression After PSA Elevation Following Radical Prostatectomy." The title of the article from the medical journal is appropriately negative, implying that cancer often does reappear after surgery. It was difficult for me to see how this information could possibly warrant the positive title (Relief To Cancer Patients) in any media.

Before reviewing this data, it is important to put the essence of the JAMA title in perspective. This requires thinking back to when the decision to have a radical prostatectomy (surgery), instead of radiation or one of the several non-conventional treatments, among which was "to do nothing." As long as you were not too old (below 70), and were in good enough condition to withstand the operation, surgery would likely be touted as the "golden alternative"—the only treatment that could totally rid your body of cancer cells. It was strongly "implied" that those who could meet the requirements to qualify for surgery were fortunate, because removing the prostate (surgery) would remove the cancer—the implication being that there would be no cancer cells left to multiply.

Now along comes these significant, and probably valid research results, informing patients what their prospects for survival are when they have opted for surgery, and cancer returns. The research is based on 1,997 men who had undergone radical prostatectomy for "clinically localized prostate cancer" by a single surgeon, at the Johns Hopkins Hospital in Baltimore between 1982 and 1997. All of these patients had experienced similar tests; PSA, digital exams, biopsies and Gleason ratings, to determine the treatment needed.

This research was presumably noteworthy because so many patients received the same treatment, both before and after surgery, performed by a single surgeon at the same location, which made it possible to maintain and control records and follow through for a reasonable number of years.

The objective of this research was to "characterize the time course of disease progression in men with biochemical recurrence after radical prostatectomy"—because about 35% of surgery patients, historically, experience detectable PSA elevation within 10 years following surgery.

Since the surgery on the patients in this test occurred during a 15-year period, the consequences of treatment were less known for the patients treated more recently. However, because of the commonality of the group, it was scientifically feasible to extrapolate the findings from the early patients to predict the outcome of the later ones. Here are some of the conclusions derived from this extensive research:

No man experienced recurrence of cancer with an undetectable serum PSA level.

Between 27% and 53% of men will experience a detectable serum PSA elevation within 10 years following surgery.

The longer the interval is between surgery and PSA elevation, the longer will be the interval from PSA elevation to cancer metastasis.

The likelihood of having an undetectable PSA level at 10 to 15 years after surgery are predictable based on the level of pretreatment PSA, pathologic and Gleason readings.

23% of the men who demonstrated a PSA elevation had an undetectable level for five years. 4% were undetectable for 10 years prior to recurrence. This invalidates the theory that when you go five years without recurrence, you're home free.

The risk of developing metastatic disease (cancer tumors) after PSA elevation was shown to increase in relationship to the level of the Gleason score. Men with Gleason scores of 7 or lower had a 73% chance of remaining free from progression at 5 years. Those with Gleason scores of 8 and over had a 40% chance of a 5-year interval.

Men who progressed to recurrence of metastasis within 1 to 3 years following surgery died due to cancer at a higher rate than those men who developed metastasis at 4 to 7 or more years after surgery.

There was an 82% metastasis free survival at 15 years following surgery of all the men in this study group.

This study, as in many others, indicates that once metastasis recurs after surgery, the application of non-curative therapies (referred to as salvage treatment) don't impact the eventual outcome.

24

PSA ELEVATION SCARE

❦

(June 99)

A month or so after I had studied this research, I was due for another PSA test and an appointment with my Urologist. When I asked him what he got out of this Johns Hopkins study, he thought for a few seconds and said that it seems to be quite apparent that once cancer comes back after surgery, most of the follow-up tests and treatments that are often provided are probably unnecessary. Unfortunately for recurring prostate cancer patients, I think he got the right message. This part of the study reminded me of the large group of men in my support group who were all on (probably useless) salvage treatment.

Since I completed my Radiation therapy in August of 1997 I had undergone three PSA tests, and the reading each time had been at the very low level of 0.2. This consistent reading had been very comforting, because the PSA level was the single indicator of my cancer status. If it stayed static, I was OK. If it increased, a problem was rearing its ugly head.

As usual, six months had elapsed much too quickly. As the June, 1999 date for my 4th post-surgery PSA test approached, I was becoming increasingly apprehensive. My blood was drawn 10 days before my appointment with my urologist. When I walked into his office, I asked the receptionist for a copy of the test. There it was, staring out at me—a reading of 0.3—an elevation of 0.1. My stomach turned to stone and I could feel blood rushing to my face.

When Dr. Callon read the test results to me, he picked up on my somber reaction and cautioned me against reading too much into it, reminding me how slow moving PC is and how long it took to move up just one tenth of a point. I realized that there wasn't much else he could say, but I wasn't consoled. There was no advice dispensed about anything I could do. So by not consoling me in any way, he had just confirmed my own assumption that I was in trouble.

Realizing that the Hopkins research of 1,997 men, which I had studied, dealt exclusively with surgery patients, I asked Dr. Callon how he thought the results would have compared with a study of the same number of radiation patients. He responded that there could be no comparison. **He explained that in surgery, all the cancer should have been removed.** So if a detectable PSA level returned, the purpose of the surgery had failed. However, **in Radiation, all of the cancer is not removed—it is merely reduced, damaged or put into remission.** Since remnants of cancer cells usually stay in the system, there is likely going to be some measure of PSA remaining in the system. Given enough time, it will eventually reappear, hopefully not soon enough to be the cause of death.

During this little discussion, my mind flashed back to 1997 when I reluctantly made the decision to undergo radiation treatments. I'm pretty sure that I wasn't told that after 38 radiation treatments, some cancer cells would more than likely survive and that if they did, they would most certainly continue to grow and multiply. In fact, I recall that I was encouraged to feel that if my cancer was confined to the prostate, which I believed it was, radiation would eliminate it just as effectively as would surgery, and without the risk of a heart attack on the operating table. In fact, it was this assurance that was most compelling in influencing me to favor radiation over surgery (plus the fact that I really didn't have a choice). And then to be told, two years later, that radiation usually leaves some cancer cells alive, to grow and multiply, albeit slowly, was disheartening, to say the least.

This obviously was a substantial setback and took its toll on my morale for several weeks. My hope, of course, was that the PSA test was flawed, and that the next test would be back to 0.2. If not, the most I could hope for would be for the very slowest rate of elevation in the time spans between PSA tests. If the PSA would continue to elevate slowly enough, my normal life span might very well win the race.

In August 1999, I was informed that the "Man To Man" support group that I had attended in 1997 had a new facilitator (leader). Since I had quit going only because I disagreed with the philosophy of the facilitator, I arranged to go to the next monthly meeting. The meeting turned out to be very beneficial. There were two nuclear medicine specialists on the program who provided information on searching the Internet for useful information. They also shared a newsletter with us from a 55-year-old Urologist who had his PSA tested for the first time and discovered that he had prostate cancer—he had a PSA of 20. He had established a Prostate Forum, in the form of a newsletter, which he puts out monthly, which is like a journal in that he walks his readers through each treatment decision he makes, along with the reasoning that went into each decision. By his own admission, he has deviated from some of the recommendations he had previously made to his patients. I couldn't help but think what a great Urologist this patient will be if he would survive this ordeal.

With a PSA of 20 and a Gleason of 7, he was acutely concerned that the cancer had spread beyond the prostate. I learned that he utilized a relatively new treatment called the ProstaScint Scan, which had only become available within the last two years. It was supposed to be considerably more sensitive than an MRI in its ability to detect the location of cancer cells. Even so, when it was used to detect cancer in lymph nodes, it was effective about 70 to 80% of the time versus 20 to 30 % of the time with a CAT scan. Also, this process was time-consuming, arduous and expensive. He finally had his lymph nodes removed, just to be sure, and learned that they could detect no cancer. However he was quite certain that cancer had penetrated the prostate capsule (based on his PSA and Gleason scores) and invaded the tissue surrounding the gland which eliminated surgery as an option. In the final analysis, he chose a combination of hormonal therapy, external-beam radiation and radioactive-seed implantation.

When the question and answer session started, I directed my question to the principal doctor. I explained that for two years after radiation, my PSA had held at 0.2 and that it had recently elevated to 0.3. How concerned should I be? He explained that this elevation would indicate that a live cancer cell was in my system, and that it wouldn't necessarily be in the prostate. It could be anywhere, even in the lymph nodes. During the meeting he had described a relatively new "ProstaScint Scan" devise that has proven to be the best method to use to visualize the location of cancer cells. He suggested that this might be something to consider. When I left that meeting, I was numb with renewed concern about my elevated PSA and the necessity to do something, rather than to routinely wait for six months for my next blood test.

Soon after I attended that support meeting and three months after my elevated PSA test, I decided to take some action. I realized that I was doing a lot of worrying that wasn't very healthy, and maybe it wasn't even justified. In addition, I felt the need to get some of the load off of my back and share it with someone else. So I called my Radiologist, Dr. Bruce, and asked for a consultation. His nurse called and asked me to pick up a prescription and get blood drawn for another PSA test, and to come in three days later, which would allow time for them to have the test results.

Dr. Bruce came in, went through the usual digital exam of my prostate, allowed me to get dressed, and then he handed me a copy of the test results. When I saw that test score of 0.2, I could hardly believe my eyes. It wasn't elevated after all. All of my worrying had been for naught. In that instant, I believe I experienced what a man feels the moment he is released from prison. This certainly was confirmation that sometimes it pays to take things into your own hands.

Dr. Bruce explained that even though the PSA is the best available test for PC right now, it is far from precise. For one thing, the presence of PSA is measured in nanograms. A nanogram is one billionth of a gram. Attempting to get an accurate measurement of something that minuscule would be difficult. Measuring the difference between a reading of 0.2 and 0.3 would seem to be even more difficult. In addition, there are a variety of things that a prostate might react to that can result in a false and inflated reading. Almost anything that has recently applied any physical pressure to the prostate gland, such as a digital rectum exam by a doctor, or to have just ridden a horse or a bike, any one of these could cause an elevated, thus a false, reading. Even trying too hard to have a bowl movement just before leaving blood might result in a reading that is false, as can having ejaculated the night before. In fact, the doctor described an unusual incident where a patient's last PSA was 2.5, which wasn't much more than he had tested for the past year or so. So when his next PSA registered a six, it was unbelievable and it just couldn't be right. After questioning his patient intensely, he finally admitted that a few days before the test, he had fallen from a building and landed astraddle a wood fence, resulting in extreme pain and bruises to his groin area. He had even kept this accident a secret from his wife because he wasn't supposed to have been on the building in the first place.

Dr. Bruce admitted that there were many things doctors don't know about cancer and about PSA tests. But in his judgment, all PSA readings of less than 0.5 are negligible, and the differentials among such small numbers are meaningless.

When I left that office, I felt that I had received accurate advice and council. As young as he is, Dr. Bruce is very bright and has a tremendous amount of knowledge. And in addition, it is obvious that he has genuine concern and compassion for his patients. When leaving his office, I never had the feeling that he was anxious for me to leave so he could hurry to another patient, as is so often the case with some doctors.

As I reflect back on that experience with my PSA elevation, I really am irritated that I spent three months being unnecessarily despondent. It is amazing how one doctor can be so much more comforting than another when the information they have about a mutual client is the same. I wonder if those specialists at the support group meeting, who added fuel to my already heightened concern about my 0.1 elevation, were looking for another customer to help finance their expensive machine.

It was on the 15th of December 1999 when one of our closer friends, Don, was entered into one of the better "assisted living" facilities in our town. He had been living by himself ever since his wife had died about six or seven years prior. More recently prostate cancer had been detected and he had chosen to have radiation seed implantation as opposed to external beam radiation. His urologist, as well as a radiologist, had recommended seed implantation so enthusiastically that, after his first consultation, he made an appointment for the treatment. His explanation was that he was so impressed with this urologist that he would feel comfortable following his advice. Unfortunately, when the treatment was finished, he had lost his bladder control, and even several weeks later, he still had to use a catheter and a bag to retain the urine. In the meantime he had been extremely uncomfortable and disappointed that the results of the treatment were so far different from what he had been led to believe it would be. During the course of this experience, even before the treatment, Don had begun to be forgetful, and from time to time seemed to be "in another world" for short periods of time. The fact that he got progressively worse after the radiation treatment could very well be associated with being anesthetized, or from some other aspect of the treatment. He was scheduled for a series of tests to attempt to determine what was causing his psychological problem. In addition, he indicated that they were thinking of going back into his prostate area to see if there was a way to alleviate the incontinency problem

After I learned about Don's urination problem I found out that his hospital had only been doing seed implantation for nine months—contrasted with the University of Pittsburgh Hospital, for example, where it has been practiced for six or seven years at least. I had learned from my prior study that the success of this procedure hinges directly upon how precisely the seeds are implanted—and that this expertise comes largely from experience. I'm just thankful that after I had researched seed implants as an alternative treatment, I decided against it primarily because there hadn't been enough time yet to verify its long-term results. This case certainly brings in to question its short-term results as well. Several months later it was determined that the psychological problem Don was suffering from was the early stages of Dementia and may have had nothing to do with his prostate treatment experience.

Some news about a new method of treating cancer was contained in a pamphlet from our major hospital recently that caught my interest. This method involves "customized" immunotherapy of cancer. "Instead of impairing the body's immune system, as chemotherapy ends up doing, immunotherapy boosts the defenses, activates immune function and enhances its ability to destroy tumors. The underlying principle of this research is simple. Each individual tumor is unique to that person; similar to fingerprints or DNA. Using this approach, the initial treatment for a patient with breast cancer, for example, would be surgical removal of her tumor. A portion of the tumor would then be processed to obtain her own heat-shock proteins, which would be saved in the freezer. Should the cancer return or spread to other parts of her body, she would receive immunotherapy using her own heat-shock proteins. These proteins, injected into the skin, would activate the body's defenses to fight the cancer and destroy the tumor."

"This customized immune therapy would be well tolerated and have no side effects because it would come from cells of the same person to whom it would now be administered."

25

DOCTOR-PATIENT RELATIONSHIP

A recent study revealed that "in nine out of ten decisions made between doctor and patient in routine office visits, the doctor did not discuss the issue enough to allow the patient to make an informed choice. Primary care physicians frequently made decisions without discussing the intervention with the patient or seeking their involvement." This was reported in the Journal of the American Medical Association. Hopefully doctors will respond favorably to this criticism.

Of course there are frequent cases, such as an inflamed appendix, when there aren't a number of alternatives—that organ needs to be removed, and there would be little need to discuss alternatives. However, in many cases in my experience I would like to have had the doctors take more time to explain the diagnosis in language I could understand and to describe alternative treatments in more detail. The doctors who do this very well establish a bond with a patient that is most desirable. Doctors also enhance this process when they draw pictures of the problem. An example would be a sketch to show the blockage in an artery to the heart and how the bypass would solve the problem. Surely most patients would feel more comfortable and confident when they understand the problem and when the explanation of the solution makes sense.

I have no idea how doctors are trained in medical school about relating to their patients. When they start to practice they are probably more idealistic in their doctor-patient relationships than they will be later. Also, each patient is different and so the interaction would change from patient to patient.

It has been my experience that a patient can have a lot to do with the relationship that gets established with a doctor. As a matter of fact, getting the proper medical attention needs to be a working partnership between the doctor and the patient. Patients should be appropriately assertive about what they expect from the doctor. They should spend some time before an appointment to prepare, by writing down the important questions they want answered. Just as a doctor is expected to review your file before he comes in to greet you, you also should have prepared. Obviously any symptoms you have been experiencing should be part of your notes. Anticipate the questions he usually asks and prepare for them in advance so you don't have to answer on the spur of the moment—maybe forgetting something significant.

I know men and women my age who hold doctors in such awe that the communication process between them is inhibited. One couple I know, by their own admission, refrain from telling their doctor about minor aches and pains, even when they are in his office. These same friends are also overly considerate about bothering to call a doctor when they have a problem because "they are so busy I hate to bother them." This type of relationship is not only detrimental to the patient's welfare, but it obviously deprives the doctor from providing optimum care.

At the end of March 2000, I met with my urologist to review my PSA results six months after my test results had dropped from 0.3 to 0.2. This time, when I was told that my PSA had elevated to 0.4, actually doubled, I took it in stride. I guess I had accepted the lesson from my September visit with Dr. Bruce, who convinced me that a variable of a few tenths is relatively immaterial, considering the miniscule measurements in nanograms. But knowing me, as the time for another test draws near, I'm afraid my apprehension will begin to rise.

Our local newspaper recently ran an interesting series on the progress of alternative medicines in the past decade and its influence in the market place and in the doctor's offices. Dr. Andrew Weil, a Harvard-educated physician, turned healthcare practitioner, helped trigger an explosion in the growth of health food stores when he wrote "Spontaneous Healing" in 1995. About the same time, congress deregulated nutritional supplements, allowing manufacturers to broaden their claims without governmental scrutiny or control (in contrast to prescription drugs).

The medical fraternity was awakened in 1997 when a survey revealed that more people were visiting alternative caregivers than were visiting doctors; 629,000 versus 386,000.

I think there is potential value to be derived from certain foods and supplements, and the medical profession is, finally, beginning to join the effort to get the necessary research done. This is particularly critical in the area of fortifying the immune system. The foods we select to eat can substantially contribute to this effort. It shouldn't be that difficult to run tests to validate the comparative value of foods and to measure their contribution to the immune system, but it will take many years. It is a reasonable project to not only start, but to accelerate, so that our children might experience the benefit.

26

GENETICS PLAY A ROLE

In July 2000, the Associated Press, followed quickly by the major weekly magazines, reported that heredity accounts for many cancer cases. This study was done in Scandinavia and they utilized the history of 89,576 twins to get reliable enough statistics to analyze 11 types of cancer. Their findings concluded that genes account for 42 percent of the risk of prostate cancer, 35 percent of the risk of colorectal cancer and in breast cancer, 27 percent. For other types of cancer, the genetic risk is lower.

This is extremely new research and has yet to survive the response of the scientific skeptics, but genetics has always been a known factor for cancer. It is just that these percentages are considerably higher than figures that have been used in the past. At the same time, there was nothing in this study to dispute the contribution to cancer caused by the environment. Factors like what we eat, drink, breath and smoke, how we live and what chemicals we are exposed to seemingly account for roughly twice the risk of cancer that genetics do. At the same time, if your genetic history increases your susceptibility to cancer, it would be a red flag that should prompt you to take precautions in a number of ways, including more frequent testing.

Our son, Greg, has just turned 51. His first PSA tested 0.4 three years ago and recently tested 0.4. This seems to be about average for his age. I have made certain that he realizes the need to get retested every few years. He also knows that a significant change in a reading is more important than the score itself.

Unfortunately genetics play a substantial role between father and son regarding susceptibility to prostate cancer. I had never given much thought to the possibility that my having prostate cancer might some day directly endanger my son—but apparently it is in the process of occurring and it makes me extremely uncomfortable. Hopefully, before he is 65, I feel quite confident now that one of the dozens of potential remedies on the medical horizon will be available for him.

The baby boomers, now into their 50's, need to realize that they are vulnerable to this disease whether or not there is a genetic factor. The two most critical life-saving facts they must be aware of are:

1. There are no early warning signs (like pain) to let them know that cancer cells are active in their bodies.

2. The only way to detect the presence of prostate cancer is to have a digital exam and a PSA test.

3. Only when PC is detected at an early stage (when it is confined to the prostate) is there a reasonable chance that it can be successfully treated.

Hopefully, we are now moving into a period when more money and attention is accelerating prostate cancer research, and there are literally dozens of promising efforts in various stages of testing. The fact that it will still take a number of years to bring the first of these experiments to fruition and then get FDA approval only emphasizes the need for baby boomers to be alert about the present danger. The first PSA test should be taken at least by age 50, and maybe sooner. How that test measures can then be the guide to the schedule for the next one. Taking this seriously and responding to a few simple guidelines can, and probably will, be the difference between life and death.

I recently had discouraging news from my friend Gary, who had his prostate removed in February 1999. During the after surgery biopsy, the pathologist had discovered a hole in a capsule from which a cancer cell could have escaped. The implication would be that a cancer cell could already be in the bloodstream out of the confines of the prostate. Once the cancer cell escapes into the bloodstream, it would grow more rapidly. Gary told me that each PSA test through April, 2000 had registered 0.1. Then he was tested in mid-July and had a PSA of 0.3. He knew he was in trouble. He was referred to a radiologist who recommended radiation as well as about four months of hormonal treatment. In the meantime they were testing him each month and the reading through October 2000 had held at 0.3.

Gary had made arrangements for a second opinion from a renowned specialist at Duke University Hospital who agreed with the local radiologist. 40 radiation treatments were then applied in early 2001, along with hormonal treatments which to be continued for two years. A year later Gary is still having to put up with the discomfort of the nightly hormonal sweating, but his PSA tests are staying at below 0.1, which is encouraging. As near as I can determine, it isn't common for a 59 year old man with a low PSA reading to have to undergo three treatments consecutively. But hopefully, now he can start getting on with his life.

27

THE LAST CHAPTER

I n 1975, when I was diagnosed with a heart problem and was told that I would need a by-pass operation, I was shocked and nervous having to deal with something I knew nothing about. Fortunately, an acquaintance where I worked heard about my problem and came into my office for a visit. He explained that he had undergone such an operation and proceeded to explain exactly how it would be performed and how it had been a lifesaver for him. I will never forget how helpful this visit was and how much more comfortable I was when the time came for my heart operation.

In 1997 when I received a positive biopsy for prostate cancer, I was also shocked and nervous. But an additional disheartening problem was having the personal responsibility to make sure that I would select the best possible treatment. This was extremely difficult since I knew nothing about the subject nor did I know anyone who had experienced prostate cancer. It was during the early stages of this frustration, when I was frantically searching for information that would help me make a treatment decision, that I began to think of writing the kind of book that I wanted, but couldn't find. In this way, I felt that I would be helping those coming after me. I decided to write it like a journal, just as it was happening, along with pertinent information about prostate cancer that I would be discovering in my research. I felt also that it would be of some value to share my emotional ups and downs that I would be experiencing along the way. So that is what I have attempted to do.

As time went by I began to realize that I would need to decide when to bring this book to a close. During the course of this experience I read a book written in journal form by a man who was dying of cancer (not prostate). Near the end he died, and the final chapters were written by his wife. I decided I would like to write this last chapter myself.

I started this book even before I finished my radiation treatments, which was on August 8, 1997. As I am typing these final words, it is in the spring of 2002. My first PSA test result in September, 1997 measured 0.22. Over four years and eight tests later it measures 0.2. At this last test, my radiologist gave me an A+ and declared that annual tests by my urologist from now on would be sufficient (instead of every 6 months). I walked out of his office feeling pretty good. With no PSA elevation in over 4 years, any future elevation would likely be equally slow in developing cancer cells soon enough to affect my life span. At 77, although I will need to continue PC check-ups, I'm thankful for the success of the treatment I chose and I'm optimistic about the future.

My purpose for writing this book has not been to give advice to others. It has been to share with you my experiences in a very candid and open way. I tried to reflect my emotions as I reacted to experiences and discoveries. I searched deeply for applicable medical test results that would help to better know what to expect, feeling that statistics would be more reliable than words. I tried to put what I learned in a language that would be understood. I also included my experiences with friends and acquaintances along the way, who were battling PC, some winning and some not.

During the over four years between starting and ending my account, there has been an upsurge of promising medical discoveries pertaining to treatment, and even prevention, of prostate cancer. Some are already in early stages of development and testing in research centers. Hopefully, within the next decade, some of these discoveries will hit the jackpot.

A recent research report concerning prostate cancer patient's relationships with their physicians stated the following: Almost all physicians reported that they discuss treatment options—yet one in six men surveyed don't recall the discussions. Even worse, regarding having discussions about the effect of PC treatment on the quality of life, one third of the patients disputed having the discussion with their physician.

Just as doctors need to communicate well with patients, so do patients need to relate effectively with their doctors. Doctors need all the help they can get from the patient in order to make the best diagnosis. Patients need to understand and follow instructions of their doctors. Good health is at stake in both instances.

So finally, here are some suggestions to both doctors and patients to enhance the relationship that will help to foster better health.

SUGGESTIONS TO DOCTORS

- Take time to review test results with patients and give them a copy to take home. This allows the patient to evaluate progress or regression, and the spouse to know what is going on. Very few men I have asked remember what their last PSA or cholesterol test score was.

- Radiologists should advise patients to avoid taking vitamins and supplements during treatments because they will work against the radiation that is being applied specifically to destroy cells. Most patients I have talked to take supplements of some kind.

- Urologists, or someone in their office, should take sufficient time to familiarize patients with treatment options that are available. The explanations should be accompanied with updated written material. This would allow the patient to study and evaluate before making a decision.

- Neither urologists or radiologists should arbitrarily set 70 as the age that determines whether you should have radiation as opposed to surgery. Many patients who are 72 are in better condition to withstand surgery than other patients who are 65.

- Recent research indicates that over 90% of the time a treatment is being determined, urologists recommend surgery and radiologists recommend radiation. This would seem to indicate that the best interests of the patient is not always being applied. This would also magnify the necessity for the patient to actively participate in making the treatment decision.

- The biopsy report from the pathologist should best be reviewed again with the patient several days after the initial shock of a positive biopsy. It should be discussed thoroughly enough so that the implications of the Gleason rating is understood (it projects the aggressiveness of the cancer). A copy should be provided to the patient so it can be shared with the spouse.

- I would advise specialists to share the most current statistics pertaining to the likely success or failure of each treatment. This needs to be the most reliable information available. It should be reviewed and provided in written form.

- The risk of side effects that might occur should be candidly discussed, especially those with long-term consequences such as incontinence and impotence.

- Ideally, urologists would provide prostate cancer patients with a book containing all the up-to-date information that a patient would need to know. Until then, they should provide much more written information than they do.

- Doctors need to take the necessary time and effort to be sure that the patient fully understands information and instructions.

SUGGESTIONS TO PATIENTS:

- Take plenty of time and utilize all the resources at your disposal in selecting your specialist. Put more weight on experience than on personality alone.

- Don't be hesitant to challenge your doctor when you don't understand complicated information and instructions. If you don't understand, tell him you don't understand—or ask him to write it down.

- Be bold enough to change doctors who have proven to be ineffective, or who aren't sensitive to your needs. Life is too short to do otherwise.

- Take the time to do some research on your own in order to better assess the decisions that will be made. Support groups can be a useful resource (American Cancer Society's Man to Man, just for prostate cancer, is available in most large cities.

- Try to establish a partnership with your specialist. Be sure to keep him advised of any symptoms you are experiencing even if they are minor. Then ask him to be candid about your progress, or lack of progress. You have a right to feel confident that he is providing the proper treatment.

- Between visits, write down questions or problems you are experiencing as they occur so you can be specific as to time and duration. Take the list on your next visit.

- Be sure to provide your doctor with an updated report on what medication you are taking, including over-the-counter vitamins. This is frequently neglected.

- Don't deviate from following the doctor's instructions about taking his prescribed medication, or OTC medicine, without checking back with him first.

- Research on your own, using current publications, attending seminars provided by hospitals, and searching the Internet.

- Recognize that some of our health problems occur because of genetics and family history, which we can't control. But lifestyle changes can often impact our health and longevity to a far greater degree than treatments by our doctors. The most common choices, such as smoking, gaining excess weight, not exercising, not eating nutritious food or over eating, are all contributors to serious health problems. And all are usually controllable by change in your lifestyle.

- And above all, actively participate in the decisions that affect your health care—you have the right and the obligation to yourself to do so.

- And finally, once you have established your healthy living routine and have made the best choices you can make, spend more time doing what you enjoy doing. An optimistic attitude can contribute to your health.

ABOUT THE AUTHOR

Stanley K. Sandage grew up on a farm in southern Iowa during the "great depression." He served in General Patton's Third Army in WWII as a sergeant in a machine-gun platoon. He fought in the 65th Infantry Division in campaigns in Germany and Austria, earning a Bronze Star medal and the Combat Infantry Badge.

Stan is a graduate of Drake University and is retired from a management career with the B. F. Goodrich Company. He is the author of The Horse That Wouldn't Die, 1996, and a contributing author of Wordspinners of the Akron Manuscript Club, 2001. He is currently editing a semi-annual magazine for his world war II Division Association.

Stan and his wife Peggy live in Akron Ohio. They have two children, Greg and Susan, and six grandchildren.

0-595-23510-7

www.ingramcontent.com/pod-product-compliance
Lightning Source LLC
Chambersburg PA
CBHW061315280526
45784CB00002B/992